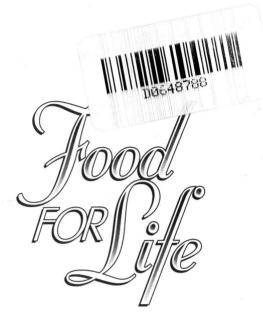

Food
FOR Life

Food FOR Life

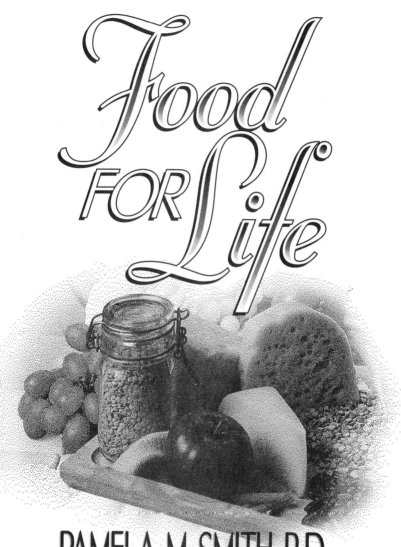

PAMELA M. SMITH, R.D.

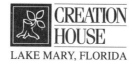

CREATION HOUSE
LAKE MARY, FLORIDA

FOOD FOR LIFE by Pamela M. Smith
Published by Creation House
Strang Communications Company
600 Rinehart Road
Lake Mary, Florida 32746
Web site: http://www.creationhouse.com

Unless otherwise noted, all Scripture quotations are from the Holy Bible, New International Version. Copyright © 1973, 1978, 1984, International Bible Society. Used by permission.

Scripture quotations marked NKJV are from the New King James Version of the Bible. Copyright © 1979, 1980, 1982 by Thomas Nelson, Inc., publishers. Used by permission.

Scripture quotations marked TLB are from The Living Bible. Copyright © 1971. Used by permission of Tyndale House Publishers, Inc., Wheaton, IL 60189. All rights reserved.

(Revised edition), June 1997

8901234 RPG 98765
Printed in the United States of America

⌣ ACKNOWLEDGMENTS ∾

Special thanks and love to my husband, Larry, for his consistent love and support;

to my daughters, Danielle and Nicole, for keeping me ever focused on my priorities in life;

to my mom, Mae Martin, who never hesitates to help and never ceases to care;

to Sherry Martin and Beverly Brim, my trusted assistants, who have worked overtime to show God's love to me and to our clients;

to Carolyn Coats, who is God's very special gift to me;

to David and Caron Loveless, our dear friends who lead Discovery Church, for modeling a life of vision;

to Debbie Cole and all the staff of Creation House for going the distance in encouragement and helps as this book has been transformed;

and to all my clients and friends who, in sharing of themselves, have shaped this message.

ᕦ CONTENTS ᕤ

WHEN I COMPLETED the original manuscript for *The Food Trap*, I hoped it would shine the light of truth on eating dependencies and yo-yo dieting for those caught in a web of deception. I wanted it to be their first step to freedom.

Since then I have spoken in counseling sessions and at conferences to countless numbers of courageous souls who have seen the truth and entered the process of transformation. And I have received many wonderful, thoughtful letters from people from all walks of life, with all kinds of needs, sharing how *The Food Trap* has touched their lives. These letters tell the stories of their struggles and, often, their emancipation.

I rejoice to hear of individuals who come to value themselves and desire to walk in the purpose for which they were created. As people embrace the truth of who they are and why they've been created, they learn to live well — and nourish themselves too. They take good care of themselves, not out of duty or feelings of guilt, but out of a natural desire to be healthy and happy. And as they live well, it overflows into those around them.

Today, as I look anew at the subject of *The Food Trap*, my heart's desire is to open the door to freedom even wider. The "little" snares of life — lack of self-care, erratic eating, unhealthy choices, poor sleep patterns, no exercise — can hinder abundant living just as much as deep emotional issues can imprison so many people.

We must take our eyes off these snares and learn to live free of them. We need a new perspective on food — physical, emotional and spiritual food — that frees us to be well, keeps us well and energizes us to live fulfilled lives.

I pray that you will find this book filled with encouragement, hope, truth and practical helps to bring you greater peace, freedom and fulfillment.

Special blessings,
Pam

LIVING LIFE
ON THE
FAST TRACK

E NERGY THAT LASTS as long as our days do. Sharpened concentration, enduring memory, high productivity. Bright attitude, a hopeful perspective, stress resiliency. This is the "right stuff" for living life.

We dream of feeling great. We long to feel better. We read about it. We talk about it. But do we really live it?

Nope — at least, many of us do not. A life filled with wellness has become an elusive butterfly. Strides toward wellness are typically only attempts at dieting — with failure as the result. Diets begin, and diets end. Most people don't make it through the first week, let alone the first month.

The bottom line is that most of us don't need to learn how to diet or control disease; we need to learn how to eat for life.

Throughout my years of counseling, people have come to me seeking a quality of life filled with energy and well-being. Some people also knock on my door because they want to lose weight. Some need only to trim down to a more fit shape. (They have the "furniture disease" — their chests have gone to their drawers!) Some need to manage stress better. Some desire more energy. Others come very ill, needing a nutritional plan to control serious diseases.

Early in my practice I sensed that most of my clients needed simple nutritional education. Rather than finding out what they shouldn't eat, they needed to learn what they should eat, when to eat and how to balance their intake in such a way to benefit their bodies.

My clients needed to learn how to break away from the typical American eating style while still living a normal lifestyle. And they needed to learn the vital part food plays in their well-being.

As they put this education into practice, many succeeded in achieving their wellness goals — more energy, leaner bodies, lower cholesterol or stress resiliency — and have maintained those goals as a way of life.

Many embrace a new way of life, but not *all* do. A good number of people come seeking to make genuine change, but their resolutions fall short when it comes to follow-through. I have discovered that education alone, even solid truth, is not enough. Information does not change lives. Only revelation provides lasting change.

Information can be received as head knowledge and may give momentary inspiration, but revelation is received into the heart. It fuels long-lasting motivation and outperforms a good idea or something we "should" do. We change our way of eating when we see — truly see — the difference it makes in our personal lives.

I have also discovered through my sixteen years of practice that eating well is not enough to make us well. It is clear: There is more to living well than caring for and feeding our physical beings. We also have to care for and feed our souls—with the right kind of soul food.

Sound simple? Maybe. Is it easy? No.

Clients from every walk of life — top executives, professional athletes, homemakers, ministers, college students, teachers, retirees — have a similar plea: "I am out of energy and out of control of this thing called life, especially my eating and my health!"

Some are caught in what I coined the "food trap" — ensnared by food, overeating, dieting and the scale. Others, because they haven't taken care of themselves, are simply underfed and underfueled. They push their bodies through the day without food as though they were pushing a car down the road without gasoline. They are overcome by the stresses of life and are too busy or too tired to do anything about it.

I hear it every day: "Take care of myself? Eat well? Exercise? Relax? Pam, I have too much to do and never enough time to do it all. I surely don't have anything left over for those things!"

Truth? Well, I don't think it's the whole truth.

What we're lacking isn't the time; it's the energy. Sure, most of us are busier than we've ever been. But the problem comes when free time arises and we're just too exhausted to do anything we'd like to do or feel called to do. Instead we fall asleep on the couch, zone out in front of the TV or take part in activities or conversations that profit little.

Why? Because the things we like to do require a supply of energy we can't seem to muster up when we need it.

Energy has become a precious commodity.

An Energy Crisis

Where did all our energy go?

In the 1980s my counseling had a strong weight-and-disease-control dynamic. Now I work with just as many people who are simply seeking to live better. This reads "more energy." They have great demands on their lives, but they lack the energy supply to meet those demands.

Yet each body contains a power plant capable of producing more than enough energy to do just about anything that person wants to do, and then some. But we have lifestyle blocks to our living better, and we're letting energy stores leak away unused.

So I offer this book with a word of hope: Remove the logjams to your physical health and emotional well-being, and you'll release a virtual river of abundant life and energy. Nourish yourself with the right foods at the right time and deal with what's eating you, and the healing that is scripted into every cell of your body will flow through your being. That's how we were created. Wellness is an inside-out job.

In this book you'll find answers that will allow you to break free and live well with food for life. Rather than one more minute of making do, make this your time for doing well — and live life abundantly!

∿ PART ONE ∿

HELP!

ONE

THE
PINBALL
LIFESTYLE

IT WAS HAPPENING again. The businessman sitting next to me in the airplane was asking me what kind of work I do. Actually, he was pressing the issue. Once again I was skirting the fact that I was a nutritionist. I resist telling strangers what I do; it changes the whole course of our conversation.

You can understand why, can't you?

Even the word *nutrition* conjures up all kinds of bad thoughts and vibes. And any conversation quickly dwindles into excuses for why the person isn't eating this and is eating that.

Nutrition brings to mind the word *diet* — which in my perspective is the original four-letter word. Think about it: The very word is spelled D-I-E-T, just a letter away from the word *die*. And that's how you feel when you're on a diet — as if you're going to die!

Diets aren't just about weight loss anymore. People are on diets to lower cholesterol or blood pressure; to avoid fats, meats and pesticides; to prevent cancer; to build their bodies; or simply to feel better.

Diets are all about denial — focusing on what you can't eat. The temporary deprivation they bring cries out for a sure reward. The going "on" the diet to go "off" the diet, being "good" to being "bad" and eating "legal" foods only to "cheat" leaves us exhausted, unhealthy and usually unsuccessful.

This was certainly the life of my Delta seatmate, Howard. After I finally blurted out that I was a nutritionist specializing in wellness, he let me know that he quite possibly knew more about nutrition than I did. "After all, I've been dieting for forty-eight years!" he said. I later discovered he had been on four diets since January 1, and it was then only March. He wasn't particularly heavy; he had just battled fifteen pounds for so long that the battle itself seemed to have taken on a life of its own. His cholesterol and triglyceride levels were dangerously high (269 and 425 mg), and his blood pressure was fluctuating; yet he couldn't seem to stay consistent with any kind of positive eating change.

Like Howard, I grew up with dieting as my second language. And with good reason — I inherited a tendency toward being overweight. By the time I was eleven, I had gone on my first diet, an awful grapefruit and egg diet.

Was I overweight at the time? Not really. But I was growing, and my body shape was changing. It didn't conform to the popular "Twiggy" look of the day. Add to that an unhealthy dose of fear about my family's obesity problems, and I fell headlong into the dieting trap.

I was successful in losing the weight at first. But, sadly, I was equally successful in gaining it back — always more than I had lost. It was the classic story: I lost five pounds only to gain back eight. The next year, on the next diet, I lost ten pounds and gained back fifteen. The pendulum was swinging higher and wider each year with each new diet. All the dieting was leaving me a malnourished mess, yet weighing more than I ever had. I spent half my time discouraged and depressed — and the rest of it escaping from those feelings by overeating.

I was not alone. Not then, and not now. Many of us have spent a lifetime trying to cultivate willpower and self-discipline concerning food, only to reap discouragement and hopelessness instead.

Life's Tracks and Traps

Living life in the nineties means living tough lives — financially, relationally, politically, emotionally and spiritually. How often I hear, "It's just not the eighties anymore!"

I see the world running on two unhealthy tracks for survival in these tough times. One is a chronic lack of self-care manifested in unhealthy eating, high stress levels and near-empty energy supplies. The other is an obsessive-compulsive drive for beautiful, superhuman bodies — and the belief that if our bodies are perfect, our lives will be perfect. Often we find ourselves bouncing like a pinball between the two.

Howard was caught in the first track: a lack of self-care. He didn't eat that much, and the high-fat, sugar-laden foods he loved weren't the only problems with his eating style. He had no routine for eating; it was not unusual for him to go all day with little or no food, other than an occasional doughnut grabbed at a morning meeting and a continuous intake of coffee and diet soda. He typically ate only one "meal" a day — nonstop snacking from the time he got home at night till bedtime.

Howard exemplified a classic pattern I see every day in counseling. He was an ingenious chief executive officer of a major corporation, successful in all he put his hand and mind to.

Except in the area of eating.

On our ride to Dallas he poured out his frustrations. Eating was one area of his life he believed he couldn't control.

Actually, a three-hour plane ride with Howard allowed me to

see much in his life that was out of his control, but the weight and dieting issue was the easiest for him to focus on. He was weighted down with responsibility — and hopelessness — and unable to lift himself up. He finally said, "I just feel as if I'm killing myself with food, and my dieting failures are making me crazy."

Howard was caught in a life trap, and his way of eating was the glue keeping him stuck.

TWO

MAKING
PEACE WITH
FOOD

I'M FORTY-SOMETHING AND feel as if I've been fighting a war against my body for forty-something years. I just can't lose weight and keep it off. I think I've tried every diet created. I've swallowed pills, taken shots and eaten formulated foods and powders. I've fasted and drunk protein shakes. I've prayed and been prayed for," she told me.

"First my parents and then my husband and I have spent untold amounts of money on weight-loss programs guaranteed to work.

And they do work. Actually I can lose weight quite easily, but not nearly as easily as I can gain it back!"

Katie was in my office for the first time, seeking nutritional counseling for her "weight problem." At five-foot-three she weighed 172 pounds, the most she had ever weighed. She had started dieting in junior high, and the many diets she had been on since then had only made her fatter. She would lose 30 pounds, only to gain back 35. She would lose 20 pounds and gain back 30.

Katie's most successful diet had prompted a loss of 65 pounds — down to the thinnest she had ever been. Motivated by the invitation to her twenty-year high school reunion, she had felt thin and beautiful when she walked through the door. Unfortunately, she broke the diet that night and continued eating, and overeating, the rest of the weekend. Then came a vacation, followed closely by Christmas. She gained back the entire amount within five months. That was two years ago.

Her most recent attempt at weight loss had been one of the popular liquid-protein fasting programs; she lost 45 pounds in eight weeks. But Thanksgiving arrived, and she broke the diet — for that one day. Three weeks later she sat across the desk from me. She had already gained back 19 pounds, and she looked desperate and hopeless. She couldn't face going back on the fast, nor could she face another failure.

I see people every day who desire, maybe obsessively, a thin and healthy body, but such a body seems to be an impossible dream. They have tried everything to lose weight, no matter what the cost: diets, weight-loss programs, drinks, potions, pills, spas, fasting and feasting.

How can one person go on a diet, get rid of fat and keep it off easily, while nine others like Katie and Howard get caught in a never-ending chain of disappointing diets that lead to despair and defeat?

The odds are just that overwhelming — nine to one — that people who have lost weight will gain it back within a year. In fact, the five-year follow-up records of virtually every diet program indicate that one-third to one-half of dieters gain back more weight than they lost.[1]

A lot of people have spent their lives dieting, but they weigh more now than they ever have.

Is it what they eat? Partly. Is it heredity? Yes, that's also important. But the secret to weight loss lies in something more: being set free from the dieting mind-set and embarking on a lifestyle of health.

This may not be you. Maybe you need to gain weight. But you have a metabolism that burns whatever you put in, and you stay hungry and frenzied all the time. You want to gain muscle, not fatten up, but those milk shakes and sundaes just aren't helping.

Maybe you've found out your blood pressure or your cholesterol is high, and you are at risk for serious disease. You know you need to change your eating patterns. You've been given a diet, yet you keep on eating in a self-destructive way.

Do you feel overcome by stress, yet too sick and tired to do anything about it?

Take heart. You aren't alone either. It's the American way.

Until we are ready to go beyond dieting and look at the root problem, then sickness, fatigue, lack of self-care, overeating or weight can have a powerful grip on our lives. What is the underlying problem? I believe it is our thought patterns — our perspectives about the way we live and eat.

A Sucrets Solution

Statistics show that diets never have — and never will — prevail on a long-term basis.[2] I compare going on a diet to using throat lozenges for a strep throat infection. The pain you are soothing and the redness you might be reducing are symptoms of the real problem, a dangerous infection. But it will persist until treated properly — with antibiotics.

You who are card-carrying members of the diet generation must throw out your old belief systems and learn to separate fact from fiction.

It's a tough road. We face many mixed messages. On the one hand we hear the above statistics about diets being ineffective or even making us fatter; on the other, those before-and-after pictures in advertisements look too good to pass up.

I encourage Katie and Howard — and you — to look clearly at your dieting experience. Do you see anything wrong with the picture? If you've been trying and failing for many years, it's not that you just don't have enough willpower or discipline. Have you ever considered that you're choosing the wrong way to go about it? It's not that you need to learn how to diet; instead you need to learn how to eat for life.

A Prison Made of Rice Cakes

"I have finally realized that if I'm ever going to get this weight off, I have to give up everything I love, everything that tastes good!" This was Katie's proclamation of woe; she was convinced that healthy eating meant a life filled with rice cakes.

It's not uncommon to think that if food tastes good, it's more than likely bad for you; and if it's good for you, it's going to taste and look like cardboard. It is a rice-cake mentality.

How about you? Do you feel, along with Katie, that the choice to eat nutritiously is dooming you to a nutritional dungeon? Do you think that if food tastes like plastic, it must be nutritious, and if it's flavorful, it can't possibly be good for you?

If your answer is yes to these questions, you have lots of company. In a 1990 Gallup Poll commissioned by the American Dietetic Association, 56 percent of adults surveyed said they no longer found eating pleasurable because of their worries about fats, cholesterol and calories. Nearly half said they believe the foods they like are not good for them.

The survey reveals a tremendous amount of guilt but not much action: 36 percent said they feel guilty when they eat the foods they like, knowing they are not good for them — but they eat them anyway.

Another study, completed by the National Restaurant Association in 1993, established that 87 percent of Americans clearly believed in a link between nutrition and disease, yet only 37 percent were willing to put their actions where their beliefs were. The remainder report that, when going out to eat, they are most apt to order whatever they like, even if it's unhealthy.

This is no surprise to me. I hear it every day. But it distresses me to think what mixed-up, incorrect thinking is in the world. People feel guilty about eating unhealthy, "bad" food. But their biggest nutritional mistake is not what they eat; it's what they *don't* eat. They don't choose good foods, nor do they eat the right foods in the right balance at the right time. Eating is sporadic and erratic until, driven by hunger and low blood sugars, they choose the very foods they are striving to avoid.

The key to healthy eating is having the right perspective. You have to defeat the lie that says food is boring and tasteless. Eating well is not denying yourself. It's giving yourself a precious gift. Eating well is not focusing on foods to avoid; rather it is focusing on the fresh, flavorful and fun foods that give the body energy and health — and give you better moods!

Food was created to nourish and energize us, allowing us to thrive. Food has power to repair and restore our bodies in the wear-and-tear lives we lead. Our bodies have been fashioned to use food to help us stay healthier, feel better and live longer. The nourishment process was created to be accomplished in a pleasurable way. Food is an ally, not an enemy to be feared.

✌ Are You Fighting a War With Food? ✌

- Do you make promises to control your eating but break those promises again and again?

- Do you skip meals, especially breakfast, and hope your stomach won't notice?

- Do you feel a sense of power when you skip meals?

- Do you regularly go the whole day with little or no food, yet wonder why you are sick and tired?

- Have you tried to get through the day on coffee, tea or soda?

- Do you deny the physical damage or complications caused by your eating choices?

- Are you constantly dieting or discussing food and weight loss?

- Are you driven by a desire to be thin, equating thinness with success and being in control? Do you think about life in terms of "if only" ("if only I were thinner, then I would be married...have more friends...")?

- Do you eat more, or at a more frenzied pace, when under stress?

- Have you found yourself unable to stop eating?

- Have you ever thought, I was bad today; I'll starve myself tomorrow?

- Do you binge the week before going on a diet?

- Do you consume huge quantities of food rapidly and often secretly? Do you dispose of the evidence because you are ashamed of what you've done?

- Have you eaten to the point of nausea or vomiting, or until your stomach hurts?

- Do others view your shape differently from the way you do?

- Do you feel "good" when you eat, but when you stop eating, are you overcome with feelings of guilt, remorse or self-hatred? Do you eat more to relieve those feelings?

- Do you avoid social engagements that involve eating if you are on a diet?

- Do you sometimes think eating is a hassle?

- Do you fast or drastically cut and count calories to lose weight?

- Do you have an on-a-diet, off-a-diet mentality, rather than eating moderately and wisely as the norm?

- Do you think of any food as bad or forbidden rather than simply as food?

- Do you try to lose weight to look good for someone else?

- Have you relied on diet pills or shakes or any product that promises to do the weight-loss work for you?

- Do you try to lose weight with the mind-set that when you shed unwanted pounds, you'll become a wonderful person, forgetting that you already are a wonderful person?

If you are tired of a daily food fight, let new revelation about food help you make peace with it. Here's the victory word: The war has been won! Take hold of freedom!

PART TWO

FOOD FOR THE BODY AND SOUL

THREE

NOURISHING
THE
WHOLE BEING

W E HUMANS ARE three-parted beings: body, soul and spirit. Through the body and the soul, the spirit-man interacts with the physical world.

All three parts — body, soul and spirit — have needs to be nourished. Caring for the whole being means that we do special things to develop and maintain the inherent potential and health of our physical, emotional and spiritual beings.

Many people stumble because they don't get their needs met on all three levels — spiritually, emotionally and physically. And because legitimate needs are not being met in legitimate ways, it's just a matter of time before they are met in illegitimate ways.

Many of us know that spiritually we have been set free to live abundantly. That includes the freedom to be well; yet many of us believe we are unable to cash in on the promise. We may be strong spiritually and wounded emotionally, or sick physically and well spiritually. We may have emotional wisdom, yet live in a spiritual vacuum. Or we can starve our souls and our spirits while feeding our physical bodies.

The goal is to be well and whole in body, soul and spirit. The people I see getting well — and staying well — acknowledge and care for all three.

Yet how many times do we find ourselves doing the very thing we hate? Well, here too we have company! The apostle Paul admitted that he shared our common struggle in Romans 7:15: "I do not understand what I do. For what I want to do I do not do, but what I hate I do." He then went on to identify the culprit; he was entangled in the garments of his "old man." Paul's spirit was born again; all things had become new. But his soul — his mind and emotions — was still clothed in the old.

A few pages later he wrote to the Roman Christians, "Do not conform any longer to the pattern of this world, but be transformed by the renewing of your mind" (12:2). Our souls are transformed by the renewing of our minds, which is a process, not an overnight occurrence. In our emotions and our thoughts, we have to take off the old clothes and put on the new.

This is not always easy to do, but it is possible. Expect resistance. Habits and thought patterns — the "old clothes" — that have been learned throughout a lifetime require supernatural power and patience to unlearn.

If I learn as a child that being sick is one of the most effective ways of getting attention, I will spend a lifetime falling ill or having accidents whenever I feel ignored or unloved. With my conscious mind I might say that I hate being sick and that I believe in the promise of healing. But my "old man" has not yet learned another way to feel love. Just deciding not to be sick anymore will not be the cure. It will require unlearning the old ways and receiving the love and attention that come in healthy ways.

Similarly, renewing our minds doesn't happen when we go on one more diet or try to be "good." It begins when we change our perspective about the way we live and eat. It requires an understanding of how our bodies work and what habits we have acquired, plus the revelation for lasting change.

We have to get beyond the weight issue or even the fear of disease and focus on the here and now of life. How do you feel? How much energy do you have? What logjams are blocking your total well-being?

I have a word for you: You don't have to push or drag through each day. You can have abundant life; you can take charge of your wellness, your energy level and your weight. And you can be set free from those life traps of overeating, stress, too little rest and too little exercise. You are free to be well; you need only to choose to eat well of the food that gives life. Let's see how to do that.

Free to Be Well

Before I embraced nutrition as a profession, I was handicapped in all three areas of my life. I was searching for real answers to my questions about the purpose of life — my life. I knew I was spiritually empty, but I didn't have a clue about how to get filled. And with a Scarlett O'Hara approach to dealing with emotions ("I'll think about that tomorrow!"), I was carrying a lot of emotional baggage. Food became the obvious way to fill up my vacuums; it was also the fuel I needed to carry the emotional burden. So I was trapped — emotionally, spiritually and physically.

I was a senior at Florida State University. It was my last semester, and I was anxious to graduate and take on the world of fashion merchandising. I needed a class to fill a core requirement for my chosen field and stumbled on one in nutrition. I was on one of my many diets at the time — a severe high-protein, low-carbohydrate, lose-five-pounds-in-five-days-for-a-weekend-beach-party crash diet. I was amazed when I learned about the damage I was doing to my body by my ignorance and drive for thinness at any cost. I was paying a high price — with poor health, mood swings and a body that was sometimes fat and sometimes lean.

After an emotional seesaw and much deliberation, I changed my major to nutrition, adding such courses as organic chemistry and microbiology. That decision changed my life. At least, it changed part of my life.

As I learned more about nutrition and began to take care of my physical body, I became strong enough to overcome many of my unhealthy eating patterns. It would be some time before I learned about and responded to my emotional and spiritual needs. But just meeting my physical needs with the right kind of fuel gave me the ability to break free enough from food and dieting to see the gaping holes in my life.

Many of my clients see this also. As they become stronger physically, getting their bodies on an even nutritional keel, they are then free to see the deeper level of emotional and spiritual needs that hinder their health. Meeting the physical needs often provides the energy and motivation to deal with other issues.

Whatever our need of the moment — losing weight, gaining weight, controlling overeating, getting well — the goal is to learn how to get the body working for us and with us.

FOUR

FUEL
THE
POWER!

IN RECENT YEARS I have counseled many professional athletes, teaching them to "fuel the power," to be the very best they can be — to *win!* My goal is to help them operate from a point of strength physically, allowing their natural gifts and learned skills to flow freely.

I have become an avid basketball fan as I've worked with players from the Orlando Magic and the Los Angeles Clippers to achieve their peak game performance. During basketball season I often begin my mornings with reading the newspaper's sports section, eager to read any news about my players. (Who would ever have thought...?)

These players need my nutritional advice to meet the incredible energy demands of their sport. Starting players require endurance and stamina, while off-the-bench players have to be prepared to enter the game at any moment — in optimal condition. The demands peak at certain points in a game. One highly visible, critical peak occurs at the free-throw line.

Picture it: Shaquille O'Neal steps to the free-throw line to shoot. The entire stadium is filled with fans yelling, "Get it!" or "Miss it!" — depending on where the team is playing. He is surrounded by players from the opposing team "talking trash" and by his own teammates, on edge, depending on his bucket. The coaches are on the sideline, desperately wanting the point. Every stress mechanism within Shaq's powerful body goes into operation as performance anxiety builds.

Adrenaline spurts within the brain. Muscles tense. The heart races. Blood rushes to the extremities. Temperature control goes awry. Concentration fades. The ball is released, and, in a worst-case scenario, it hits the rim and bounces off — a miss. Dejected, Shaq has to shake it off and get back in the game.

My goal as nutritionist is to get the players' bodies strong and stable. Stabilizing the blood sugars and body chemistries means better control of the adrenaline — and less potential for a drop in energy and concentration when the pressure of the game heats up. More lean body tissue and proper fuel mean more strength and muscle control. Proper fluid balance keeps their bodies working for them — with fatigue down and protection from energy loss up. Then more balls go swish!

For the elite athlete, fueling the power means eating the right foods at the right time in the right balance, plus staying properly hydrated. To win consistently, they have to stay properly fit and fueled.

What About Us?

Most of us are not elite athletes, nor do we bring in the dollars and fame of a Shaquille O'Neal. Nevertheless, we all have an individual "court of life" in which we are expected to perform day by day with perfection, endurance and stamina.

We all have "fouls" committed against us, and we all step up to the "line" — emotionally, relationally, financially — surrounded by people, some for us and some against us. We have too much to do and, often, too few resources from which to pull.

It's a stressful way to live. And remember that when our bodies are entrenched in stressful times, they react.

We were created to survive physically. When we are hit with stressful situations, the survival mechanism goes fully into operation. In this mode the body becomes very protective of itself. Chemicals produced within the brain cause the body's metabolism to slow down and store fats, cholesterols and triglycerides. These become stockpiled energy for the "flight or fight" it believes is about to come.

In addition, the blood sugars fluctuate wildly, putting the body in a seek-and-find mission for quick-energy foods — not broccoli, but chocolate! The catch-22: In stressful situations, what we eat is stored more readily as fat and cholesterol. The body is being fed, overfed and fed wrongly, and it's storing, not burning. No wonder we're in the shape we're in. No wonder that 64 percent of Americans are considered overweight. No wonder that cholesterol and triglyceride levels are of such grave concern. No wonder we have no energy.

The Seven Secrets for Staying Fit, Fueled and Free!

I want to introduce you to the seven secrets for staying fit and fueled that, if used, will make your body work right. I developed this list to help clients, athletes and others embrace a lifestyle of fulfilled and effective living — to teach them to "fuel the power." It's based on meeting the body's needs with the right fuel at the right time in the right balance.

Unlike the diet designers you might have followed in the past, I emphasize *eating*: what to eat (not what to avoid), when to eat and why you need to eat it.

Remember this: *You don't need to learn how to diet; you need to learn how to eat.* These food-for-life secrets will cut through controversies and diet teachings; they will change your perspective about the place of food in your life.

Right now, changing your eating patterns may seem like just another duty or bondage. Actually, choosing to eat the right foods at the right time is choosing freedom. Rather than bind you, self-control frees you to be the real you — free from compulsive eating, compulsive dieting and body-abusive living. You can control what goes into your body, your energy level, your maximum healing ability and your own well-being. Thousands of people have done it — and you can too!

The seven food-for-life secrets are not a magic formula to follow. They are just timeless truths that show you how the body was designed to work and how you can choose food, exercise and rest to work for you, not against you.

∾ The Seven Secrets ∾
for Staying Fit, Fueled and Free!

❶ *Eating Is Better Than Starving*

- Eat Early
- Eat Often
- Eat Balanced
- Eat Lean

❷ *Water Is the Beverage of Champions*

❸ *Variety Is the Spice of Life*

❹ *Stress Is a Stretch That Makes You Snap or Makes You Strong!*

❺ *Exercise Is Vital to Well-Being*

❻ *Rest Is the Key to Recharging*

❼ *Wellness Is an Inside-Out Job*

FIVE

EATING IS BETTER THAN STARVING:

Eat Early and Eat Often

MY PROFESSION HAS allowed me to identify some common, though unhealthy, eating patterns in America. Come with me as I outline the typical American schedule on an average day.

Early morning: Most people report that they roll out of bed, stumble out of bed or fall out of bed, and some even confess to being dragged out of bed! The day starts out looking a little grim for most Americans. Rather than declaring, "What a glorious morning!" they sigh, "Is it really morning?"

Not only does the day begin with a lack of excitement for most of us, but it also begins with a lack of breakfast. Breakfast-skippers report that they have no time for breakfast — or no interest. They start out with little or no food — maybe a cup of coffee or diet soda on the run.

10:00 A.M.: Most people feel a subtle dip in energy, a little twang that says, "Any doughnuts around? Any Danishes?" Someone is always celebrating something! If they can find something, they eat it. But if nothing is available or they're too busy, another cup of coffee may get them by. If they don't drink coffee, they may have a diet soda to get that jolt of caffeine.

Lunchtime: Like breakfast, lunch is not a priority meal for most Americans. They may skip it altogether or do just fine with a burger on the run or cheese crackers from the vending machine — or maybe even something "healthy" like a salad. (Never mind the four hundred calories of blue cheese dressing; if it's a salad, it has to be good for you!)

Even if they feel a little drowsy right after lunch, almost drugged, they can push through and get a second wind. Actually, most Americans find they have pretty good energy and willpower and haven't been *that* hungry until that wonderful time of day I like to call the arsenic hour.

3:00 to 3:30 P.M. (arsenic hour): About now most people will eat anything and everything! No matter how much energy they've had, no matter how "unhungry" they've been, it all falls apart now. They whistle that little tune "Snickers is so satisfying," and the gorge begins.

However, if they're busy or no food is available, they may be able to push right through with another soda or cup of coffee — delaying arsenic hour until they get home.

Arrival home: Most of us walk in the door, do not pass "Go" and head straight to the refrigerator. While we're deciding what, oh, what to have for dinner, or while we're waiting for dinner to be served, we can eat an entire meal's worth of calories straight from the refrigerator. We have lots of "ration"alizations about eating at this time.

↵ Food "Ration"alizations ↝

- If I don't actually put food on a plate but eat straight from the containers in the refrigerator, the food doesn't count as calories. The act isn't premeditated, so I shouldn't be penalized for it.

- If I eat over the sink, those calories don't count either. Because I'm standing up, the food goes straight to my feet. It doesn't stop to be digested or absorbed, so it doesn't count against me.

- If I don't actually cut a brownie but just pick it to death, the calories certainly won't count. I burn so many calories chewing so many small bites.

- If I taste the food while I'm cooking, those calories are free. I'm just trying to feed my loved ones properly....

- If I eat food left on the plates or serving dishes while I'm cleaning off the table, that won't count either. Those calories should count against those wasteful people who didn't clean their plates!

Dinnertime: When most people sit down for dinner, they may be half full, and by the time they have finished dinner, they are very full — even stuffed. But as full as they may be, if they're typical Americans, they are probably left with a vaguely dissatisfied feeling: If I just had something sweet! Just something....

If there's nothing in the cupboard, or if they feel guilty enough about how much they've eaten, they may be able to ignore that sweet tooth.

8:30 P.M.: Many people have fallen asleep on the couch by this time. As a matter of fact, many don't know there is life after 8:30 P.M.; they sign off the air.

9:30 to 10:00 P.M.: If they've managed to stay awake past 8:30, they may settle down to watch some TV about now. A commercial comes on showing food so appealing that they can almost smell and taste it. They hear a noise coming from the kitchen but ignore it because the show's coming back on. Then the next commercial comes, and the noise starts again. This time it's too loud to ignore; they have a responsibility to check it out. So they go peeking around the corner into the kitchen. The freezer door is opening and closing, opening and closing, and a little round box of ice cream is calling out their name. It's the call of the wild. And the miracle is, a similar scene is happening all across the country.

Late every evening people hear a personal summons to the kitchen, and the typical day ends with that bowl of ice cream — or popcorn, chips or something!

The next day: They get up in the morning still full from the night before. They aren't really hungry for breakfast, aren't that interested in food in the morning and have no time to eat until about ten o'clock — when the whole process repeats itself.

Good Intentions Gone Bad

This "day in the life" shows where most of us go wrong. The typical American eats little or nothing until that unmanageable time of day when, no matter how strong he's been, how much energy he's had and how unhungry he's been, it all falls apart. During the arsenic hour, control, self-discipline and willpower slip out of one's grasp. The calories start rolling in.

How about you? What does your day look like? When do you eat? What do you eat? Where do you eat, and why?

Take the action step that follows and the five others throughout the book and see what a difference each one makes.

> **Action Step 1:** Keep a diary, for at least three days, of everything you eat and drink, the time you eat, how you are feeling and any exercise you may do, like the sample on page 41. Make a copy of the diary on pages 42 and 43 for your use here and with Action Steps 2 and 3.

◡ FOOD DIARY ◡

Your Name _Patti Martin_____ Week Beginning _August 8_____

Day	Breakfast	Lunch	Dinner	Comments & Exercise
MONDAY	Time: 8:15 bagel coffee w/cremora + 1 sugar	Time: 11:45 Wendy's chicken sandwich coffee w/cremora + 1 sugar	Time: 6:45 grilled chicken corn on cob salad with blue cheese dressing frozen yogurt iced tea	A.M. - tired & sleepy 3 P.M. - starving Night - fell asleep on couch; woke up craving sweets
	Snack: 9:45 Diet Pepsi	Snack: 3:30 Snickers 5:30 chips & dip	Snack: 10:00 frozen yogurt 2 choc. chip cookies	
TUESDAY	Time: none	Time: 1:00 cheese crackers Diet Pepsi	Time: 7:00 3 slices pizza (delivered) salad w/Italian dressing breadstick Diet Pepsi	A.M - woke up feeling sick; tired 4 P.M. - friend's birthday 8 P.M. - depressed; feel fat 11 P.M. - sick
	Snack: 10:00 Diet Pepsi	Snack: 4:00 cake + Diet Pepsi	Snack: 11:00 1 glass milk	
WEDNESDAY	Time: 6:00 corn flakes banana 2% milk coffee w/cremora and sugar	Time: 11:45 Diet Pepsi	Time: 7:30 (out to eat) lasagna broccoli salad with house dressing iced tea	6 A.M. - determined to eat better 9:30 A.M. - at meeting; sleepy 10 A.M. - guilty 12:00 - skipped lunch
	Snack: 9:30 doughnut & coffee	Snack: 2/4:00 Diet Pepsi	Snack: 9:00 juice bar	Aft. - grouchy Night - exhausted

Action Step 1: Sample

⤞ FOOD DIARY ⤝

Your Name _____ Week Beginning _____

Day	Breakfast	Lunch	Dinner	Comments & Exercise
MONDAY	Time: Snack:	Time: Snack:	Time: Snack:	
TUESDAY	Time: Snack:	Time: Snack:	Time: Snack:	
WEDNESDAY	Time: Snack:	Time: Snack:	Time: Snack:	

Day	Breakfast	Lunch	Dinner	Comments & Exercise
THURSDAY	Time: Snack:	Time: Snack:	Time: Snack:	
FRIDAY	Time: Snack:	Time: Snack:	Time: Snack:	
SATURDAY	Time: Snack:	Time: Snack:	Time: Snack:	
SUNDAY	Time: Snack:	Time: Snack:	Time: Snack:	

FOOD FOR LIFE

Losing the Battle, Winning the War!

How we eat is a sorry reflection of our lifestyles in terms of wellness. America is winning a lot of races, many that we did not bargain for: Globally, we have some of the highest rates of obesity, heart disease and certain cancers.

While our government focuses on the nation's strength as a world power, our "people power" is being robbed of energy, vitality and effective living.

Yet good health is part of our genetic heritage: Healing and repair have been encoded into every molecule in the human body. The secret is to live so as to promote that healing process rather than hinder it.

It's not the calories taken in but the calories burned that count. Our stressful nineties lifestyle has slowed our metabolic rate to a snail's pace, resulting in fats being stored rather than burned for energy. As I mentioned earlier, this "cocooning" effect is the result of constant stress demands and not nearly enough energy supply to meet the needs. The body was designed to slow itself down as a protective response to such energy deficits. As a result, erratic eating patterns keep our metabolism stuck in low gear, storing away every meal as if it were our last.

Regardless of the number of calories consumed when we do eat, the body can use only a small amount of energy, protein and nutrients quickly. The rest is thrown off as waste or stored as fat. Eating the American way robs the body of vital nutrients for the remaining twenty hours — until the next feeding frenzy. We not only go wrong in how much we eat or what we eat; we also eat entirely too much at the wrong time. The vast majority of us get most of our calories after six o'clock in the evening — too much, too late.

To activate our metabolisms and get our bodies working for us — and with us — we need to *eat*: 1) eat early, 2) eat often, 3) eat balanced and 4) eat lean.

⌣ Eat Early ∾

It was no mistake — Mom was right. You *do* need breakfast! Breakfast begins your day *well* by stabilizing body chemistries and starting the metabolism in high gear. This gives you more energy, an increased ability to concentrate and an appetite that is in control.

I always prided myself in not having to eat breakfast. No matter how out of control my eating may have been later in the day, breakfast was the one meal I could control. I liked the feeling of being "above" food, and I liked not wasting my time fixing food in the morning. Besides, I knew I would overeat later in the day, so it made sense to save calories where I could.

I was teaching nutrition at a college before I came face-to-face with the importance of eating breakfast — for me. All the information I was relaying to my students suddenly became revelation to me.

Even though I had not eaten breakfast for years, I became painfully aware that the negatives of skipping breakfast were occurring in my own life. Each morning I left home without it resulted in my operating at an energy handicap. I simply wasn't giving my body the energy supply to meet the demands placed on it. The demands continued, of course, and I met them. But I was paying the price with my moods, my inability to think clearly and my lack of energy. Inevitably I would overeat in the afternoon or evening to make up for what had been depleted, always playing a game of catch-up.

It was the first of many lessons I learned early in my profession: I had not been called to teach nutrition but to *live* nutrition.

The Breakfast Solution — Break-the-Fast!

How about you? Have you heard since you were five years old that breakfast is the most important meal of the day — yet you still skip it? Has it been information but not revelation?

Think of the body as a campfire that dies down during the night. In the morning it needs to be stoked up with wood if it's to burn vigorously again. Similarly, the body's metabolism (the rate at which you burn calories) has slowed to a resting state at night, having utilized all the easily available fuel. As you break the fast with breakfast, you meet the body's demand for an outside energy source and boost the efficiency of its metabolic system.

Skipping breakfast results in your body's turning to inside sources for energy, burning muscle mass (not fat!) for fuel. The metabolism slows down another notch, conserving itself for functioning in this disabled, starved state.

A slowed metabolism means that your body will function way below optimal levels and will more readily store whatever food, whenever it is eaten, as fat. The body simply isn't burning energy quickly enough to use the calories you've consumed — the fire has gone out. Eating most of the calories late in the day is much like dumping an armload of firewood onto a dead fire; it just sits. See any dead wood sitting atop your fire?

After a big meal, your body puts out an excess of insulin, a fat-storage hormone. Extra insulin prevents your fat cells from releasing fatty acids to be burned for energy.

Eating smaller meals more often is a lot like throwing logs on our slow-burning metabolic fires, getting them to burn better and brighter. It all starts with breakfast.

The Breakfast-Skipper Report

People skip breakfast for lots of reasons. Some people skip it to save calories; others skip it to save time. Some can't face food in the morning, and others just don't like breakfast foods. Have you ever said, "If I skip breakfast, I don't really get hungry until much later in the day. But if I eat breakfast, it starts some kind of appetite-monster, and I get hungry every few hours"? If all this sounds familiar, be assured that breakfast is not the problem; it is actually the solution.

Breakfast calories are much like a smart investment; the return is greater than the initial deposit. Dream as we might, we don't save calories by skipping breakfast. Instead, because breakfast gears up the metabolism, remaining calories from the day burn more efficiently rather than being stored as fat.

A recent Vanderbilt University study showed that overweight breakfast-skippers who started to eat breakfast lost an average of seventeen pounds in twelve weeks. Not only did eating breakfast speed up their metabolisms, but it also caused them to be less hungry the rest of the day.[1]

Do you have a time problem? Too much to do and too little time in which to do it? Breakfast does not have to be a time-*robber*; it is actually a time-*giver*. Because a smart breakfast stabilizes your blood chemistries, you will have more energy and alertness, even the ability to think more clearly. Breakfast makes you more productive and effective, allowing you to do what you do quickly — with fewer mistakes. How's that for a time investment?

Not hungry in the morning? Your body has more than likely gone through some chemical gymnastics while you've slept, and you may be awakening in a state of "morning sickness." It's not that you don't need breakfast — just the opposite. Breakfast will neutralize the body's blood sugars and stomach acids and, in turn, get you out of the disabled state.

Does breakfast *make* you hungry through the day? It should! Not only does starving in the morning slow your metabolism, but the resulting use of your own tissue for energy releases waste products into your system that temporarily depress your appetite and give you a feeling of fullness. You can continue to starve without feeling hunger for hours. Sadly, this backfires later in the day. As the Vanderbilt study pointed out, as soon as you begin to eat, the appetite really turns on, and you are set up to overeat too much, too late. Because you haven't eaten the right thing at the right time, you are apt to eat the wrong things at the wrong time.

You get hungry so soon after you have eaten breakfast because you take yourself out of the starved mode and lift up your blood sugars. What comes up *will* come down. Even with a correctly balanced breakfast your blood sugar will crest and fall within three hours or so. (That's when it's time to have a power snack!)

Do you need breakfast? Yes. Do you need to spend lots of time fixing breakfast? No. You can fix it quickly and eat it on the run if you must.

Some of my non-breakfast-food lovers start their days with a turkey sandwich or a piece of cheese pizza. The key is to have it, to have it soon (within half an hour of arising) and to have it balanced. A balanced breakfast supplies adequate carbohydrates and protein — unlike a piece of toast or a cup of coffee.

Have three different foods at breakfast: a quick, energy-starting simple carbohydrate (fruit or juice), a long-lasting complex carbohydrate (grains, cereal, bread or muffins) and a power-building protein (dairy, eggs or meats). And don't be concerned if the meals are not made up of traditional choices. Remember that the best thing for breakfast is what you will eat.

> **Action Step 2:** Eat breakfast every day, starting tomorrow morning. Use the sample breakfast diary as a guide, filling in the blank diary you copied for Action Step 1. Continue reading, but don't continue living another day without breakfast!

Get ready the night before and get up on time. If even the best-made plans get off to a late start, go out the door with a sandwich and an apple. Try these five-minute, grab-and-go breakfast beauties: low-fat cheese melted on whole grain toast with fruit; freshly fruited yogurt with a homemade muffin or cereal; or lean meat on toast. They make breakfast time-efficient and delicious!

Breakfast's Dynamic Duos

Choose one whole grain carbohydrate and one power protein, and combine these with a quick-energy fruit or juice.

Whole Grain Carbohydrates	Power Proteins
bread or toast	eggs or egg whites
English muffin	egg substitute
pancakes or waffles	all-fruit yogurt
whole grain cereal	skim milk
tortilla	low-fat or fat-free cheese
pita bread	lean meats
bagel or low-fat muffin	fat-free ricotta or
	cream cheese

For fun, fix-in-a-hurry breakfasts, turn to page 93 and wake up to sunshine.

❧ FOOD DIARY ❧

Your Name *Patti Martin*   Week Beginning *August 15*

Day	Breakfast	Lunch	Dinner	Comments & Exercise
MONDAY	Time: 6:30 A.M. *1 slice whole wheat toast* *1 oz. part-skim mozzarella (melted on toast)* *1 nectarine* *coffee with 1% milk*	Time:	Time:	*committed!*
	Snack:	Snack:	Snack:	
TUESDAY	Time: 6:40 A.M. *3/4 cup Nutri Grain Almond Raisin cereal* *1 cup 1% milk* *1/2 banana* *coffee with 1% milk*	Time:	Time:	*tired*
	Snack:	Snack:	Snack:	
WEDNESDAY	Time: 6:35 A.M. *1/2 whole wheat English muffin with 1 tsp. all-fruit jam* *8 oz. Stonyfield Farm yogurt* *coffee*	Time:	Time:	*a little hungry*
	Snack:	Snack:	Snack:	

Action Step 2: Breakfast Sample

49

◡: Eat Often :◡

As we observed in the "day in the life of" section, the arsenic hour is a personal sinking spell that's not pretty, yet happens to most people, most days. It leaves victims wondering how they'll ever make it through the rest of the afternoon.

The stresses that accumulate during arsenic hour are partly because of physical needs for food and rest and partly because of emotional needs. Adults and children alike are candidates, which explains the tension that often mounts when kids come home from school. Unfortunately, these sinking spells are not limited to sixty minutes; arsenic hour can last straight through till dinnertime. It robs us of tremendous quality time that can be invested in our families, our work, our friends and our calling.

You may not realize how much your energy, your appetite and even your moods are affected by your blood-sugar levels.

Blood sugars will normally crest and fall every three to four hours. As they begin to fall, so will your energy, your mood, your concentration and your ability to handle stress. If you've starved all day, the drop in sugar will leave you sleepy and craving sweets.

There is one thing that doesn't fall with blood sugars, and that's your appetite. As the blood sugars crash, the body responds by sending a chemical signal to the appetite control center in the brain, demanding to be fed. The signal is not requesting broccoli; it's screaming for quicker energy! The brain equates that with ice cream, chips or chocolate or whatever food happens to be your "special friend" at the moment.

Your personal sinking spells can be prevented by eating smaller amounts of food more evenly throughout the day. This starts by breaking the overnight fast with breakfast and needs to be carried on through the rest of the day with wise snacking, about every two and one-half to three hours. This will undergird your blood sugar with support and keep you operating from a place of strength.

Iron-will discipline has never controlled food intake and never will. No checklist or rigid diet plan will enable that control. Wisely chosen, wisely timed eating is much more fun and healthy.

Power-Snacking Smarts

Again, one of the biggest health mistakes some of us make is to starve throughout the day, saving up our calorie intake for the evening. This throws off the metabolism and sets us up for overeating, at arsenic hour or beyond. Instead, maintaining these smaller, more evenly spaced meals will keep the metabolism burning high and our appetites in better control.

Keep power snacks available wherever you are — in your car, your desk drawer or your briefcase. They can be as simple as fresh fruit or a box of raisins with low-fat cheese or yogurt, half a sandwich or even a trail mix of dry roasted peanuts and sunflower seeds with dried fruit.

When you don't have good choices available, you're likely to reach for an unhealthy snack or eat nothing at all. Either option sets you up for arsenic hour and beyond.

⌁ Food and Lifestyle Goals ⌁
to Stabilize Blood-Sugar Levels

1. Eat small amounts of food evenly spaced every two and one-half to three hours throughout the day to stabilize blood sugars. Timing is important to give the blood sugars support and not to overload the system at any one time, thus making it difficult to metabolize the nutrients properly. Those who are especially sensitive to blood sugar fluctuations may do well eating even more frequently — every two to two and one-half hours. Power snacking is a must! This kind of eating keeps insulin, a fat storage hormone, stabilized at lower levels in the bloodstream, which means less fat will be stored and more fat will be burned.

2. Use oat bran and other water-soluble fibers (oatmeal,

51

barley, brown rice, dried beans and peanuts) to slow absorption of natural food sugars into the bloodstream. Add oat bran to muffins and sprinkle it on cereal; serve beans as a meat alternative; have trail mix (see recipe on page 52) occasionally as a snack.

3. An hour of aerobic exercise every other day will help stabilize blood sugars by stimulating the metabolism and allowing sugars to pass through the cell walls more easily and be burned for energy.

4. Use little or no fat. There is no "good" fat, but small amounts of olive or canola oil are the best choices of oil. Avoid saturated fat.

5. Avoid any form of refined carbohydrate, such as white breads and white or enriched grains and concentrated sweets (products with high amounts of sugar in them or with sugar listed as one of the first ingredients). This form of sugar gets into the bloodstream too quickly and requires an increased production of triglycerides to transport it through the body to be used or stored for energy, as well as increased insulin load to burn it for energy.

6. Salmon, swordfish, albacore tuna, mackerel and hard shellfish (oysters, clams, mussels and scallops) are high in disease-preventing fish oils. For the greatest benefit eat them four times a week.

Keep a Log on the Fire

Remember the campfire analogy? Healthy snacking throughout the day is much like throwing wood on a fire, one log at a time, to keep it burning strong.

Your body was created to survive, and it interprets long hours without food as starvation. It will dramatically slow your metabolic rate to preserve your valuable muscle mass. Contrary to what you might think, in a starvation state your body turns first to muscle mass for energy and last to your fat stores. To metabolize calories and blood lipids efficiently and burn the fats for energy rather than muscle, feed your body the right thing at the right time.

Several small meals deposit less fat than one or two large meals do, even if you eat the same amount of the same food.

I plan my day to include three meals and two to three snacks (one mid-morning, one mid-afternoon and usually a snack at night). Planning to eat the right foods at the right times frees you of the constant battle between your appetite and your eating, lack of eating or compulsive overeating. My meal plans generally distribute the day's nutrition intake like this: 25 percent at breakfast, 25 percent at lunch and 25 percent at dinner, with the remaining 25 percent in healthy snacks throughout the day.

⌣ POWER SNACK SUGGESTIONS ∿

Here are some power snack suggestions that balance carbohydrate with protein:

- Whole grain crackers and low-fat cheese

- Fresh fruit or a small box of raisins and low-fat cheese

- Half a lean turkey sandwich

- Plain, nonfat yogurt blended with fruit or all-fruit jam, or Stonyfield Farm yogurt

- Whole grain cereal with skim milk

- Wasa bread with nonfat cream cheese and all-fruit jam

- No-oil tortilla chips with bean dip and salsa

- Rice cakes and natural peanut butter

- Popcorn sprinkled with Parmesan cheese
- Oat bran muffin with lowfat or skim milk
- Crispbread with sliced turkey and Dijon-style mustards
- Skim milk blended with frozen, unsweetened fruit and vanilla
- Trail mix (1 cup unsalted dry roasted peanuts, 1 cup unsalted dry roasted, shelled sunflower seeds and 2 cups raisins) Make it in abundance and bag into 1/4 cup portions for a whole snack.

∽ Snack Supply List ∽

Keep these snack supplies on hand. They're great when you're on the run or at the workplace since they need no refrigeration.

Complex Carbohydrates

Wasa bread
Harvest Crisp crackers
Cereal such as Raisin Squares, Ralston Muesli, Nutri Grain
 Almond Raisin, Cheerios
Guiltless Gourmet No-Oil Tortilla Chips or Baked Tostitos

Proteins

Laughing Cow Light (nonrefrigerated in round green boxes)
Weight Watchers skim milk in boxes
Natural peanut butter (2 tablespoons = 1 ounce protein)
Trail mix (includes carbohydrate)
Small pop-top cans of water-packed tuna and chicken;
 Charlie's Lunch Kit
Guiltless Gourmet bean dips (1/3 cup = 1 ounce protein)

Simple Carbohydrates

Small boxes of raisins
Dried apricots (4 = 1 fruit serving)
Whole fresh fruit (peaches, nectarines, plums, bananas, apples)
Boxes of unsweetened juices (no sugar added)
All-fruit jam such as Polaner's or Smucker's Simply Fruit

Keep in refrigerator:

Deli-sliced turkey and chicken
Low-fat string mozzarella cheese
Plain, nonfat yogurt (blend 1 tablespoon all-fruit jam into
    each 8-ounce serving) or Stonyfield Farm yogurt

And don't forget the water:

Bottled water
Evian natural spring water
Canada Dry Seltzer

Action Step 3: Plan your day to include power snacks and meals to fuel your body every two and one-half to three hours. Choose from any of the power snacks listed — and keep them wherever you are. Fill in your diary with the power snacks you selected for your own menu. It might look something like the sample on page 57.

In the next chapter we will take a look at the last two components of "Eating Is Better Than Starving" — eating balanced and eating lean.

∿ FOOD DIARY ∿

Your Name _Patti Martin_____ Week Beginning _August 22_____

Day	Breakfast	Lunch	Dinner	Comments & Exercise
MONDAY	Time: 6:30 bagel coffee with cremora + 1 sugar	Time: 11:45 tuna sandwich apple Diet Pepsi	Time: 5:30 spaghetti with meat sauce zucchini salad with Italian dressing water	9 A.M. – hungry 3 P.M. – feel good 6:30 P.M. – walked; had energy 8:30 P.M. – hungry
	Snack: 9:20 8 oz. strawberry yogurt	Snack: 2:30 1 slice bread 1 oz. turkey mustard	Snack: 8:30 1/2 c. Raisin Squares, 1/2 cup milk	
TUESDAY	Time:	Time:	Time:	
	Snack:	Snack:	Snack:	
WEDNESDAY	Time:	Time:	Time:	
	Snack:	Snack:	Snack:	

Action Step 3: Snack Sample

57

EATING IS BETTER THAN STARVING:

Eat Balanced and Eat Lean

W E HEAR A lot about balance in nutrition — balancing food groups, balancing weights, balancing fluids — but we don't hear much about balancing nutrient intake, particularly carbohydrates and proteins. Balance is more than just a pretty plate; it's getting the right foods at the right time with a carbohydrate and protein source at every meal and snack.

These two nutrients have different functions in your body. Carbohydrates are 100 percent pure energy; they are the perfect fuel for your body to burn. Fats and proteins don't burn so well. As a matter of fact, fat is the lowest-octane fuel around, even though it's packed with calories. Why? The body would rather store fat than burn it because it's already in a *storable* form. Unlike carbohydrate, fat has to go through a process of conversion to get to a *burnable* form, with only 10 percent used as energy and the rest thrown off as waste.

Protein can also be used as an energy source; 48 percent of protein may be converted to energy, and the rest will be thrown off as waste from the body. But it has too vital a function to be wasted as a fuel. The body uses protein as building blocks — comparable to the bricks that build up a house's wall. The carbohydrate you eat protects the protein you eat so it can be used for vital body-building functions. Protein is used for boosting the metabolism, keeping fluids in balance, building body muscle, and healing and fighting infections. Protein is the new you. Low-fat cheeses, lean meats, beans and skim milks and yogurts will enable your body to work better for you.

That's if all goes well. When carbohydrate is eaten alone, the body uses it like kindling on a fire. It burns brightly and quickly, but the body-building functions of protein do not take place. If protein is eaten alone, the body will burn it as fuel, wasting it as a less efficient source of energy. So be sure to eat them together. At every meal (and power snack) eat a balance of high-quality carbohydrates and lean proteins.

The diet designers of our time have taught us to "unbalance" these two nutrients, claiming that eating either all protein or all carbohydrate (depending on the diet) is the way to lose weight. Then there are the food-combining diets that say to eat all the carbohydrates you want, all the protein you want — just don't ever eat them together. Not only is this a road to diet failure, but it's also the road to poor health.

What's What

The easiest way to categorize what's what is to consider its source. Anything that comes from a plant gives carbohydrate.

Anything that comes from an animal gives protein. An exception to this rule is legumes — dried beans and peanuts. These plant foods are grown in the ground in such a way that, in addition to their carbohydrate stores, they absorb nitrogen (the essential element in protein) from the soil, thus becoming an excellent source of high-fiber protein — *and* carbohydrates.

The energy-giving carbohydrates you eat contain a wealth of fiber and nutrients necessary for your well-being. An eating plan high in fiber and complex carbohydrates is your best bet for living long and well. And contrary to what you've heard, carbohydrates are low in calories (it's what we put with them — butter, mayonnaise and dressing — that moves us into the weight-gaining territory).

Some forms of carbohydrates are digested and absorbed quite simply, allowing them to be quick-burning forms of energy. These are called simple carbohydrates and are found in fruits and crunchy vegetables. Others require more time to get into a usable form of energy; they are digested more slowly and are absorbed evenly into the system as fuel. These are called the complex carbohydrates. This form of carbohydrate is found in grains, root vegetables and legumes.

◡: Eat Balanced :◡

Your healthy goal is to choose carbohydrates in the most whole form possible to benefit from their inherent goodness — their nutrients and their fiber. This means using whole grains whenever possible: brown rice, oats, whole wheat, 100 percent whole grain breads, crackers, cereals and pastas. Eat fruits and vegetables with well-washed skins on — and choose fruit rather than the juice.

In addition, choose power-building proteins in the lowest fat forms you can. The body does not store protein, so it must be replenished frequently throughout the day, every day of our lives. Protein is much too vital to skip in the effort to lower fat intake. Just shift your focus to those proteins that are lean or, in the case of dairy, made from skim milk. You will read more about choosing low-fat versions of protein later as you learn to eat lean.

◡ SIMPLE CARBOHYDRATES ◡
FRUITS AND NONSTARCHY VEGETABLES

All fruits and fruit juices

apples, apricots, bananas, berries, cherries,
dates (unsweetened, pitted), grapefruit,
grapes, kiwis, lemons, limes, melons,
nectarines, oranges, peaches, pears, pineapple,
plums, raisins

Generally one serving of simple carbohydrate is obtained from 1/2 cup fruit, 1/2 cup fruit juice or 1/8 cup dried fruit.

Nonstarchy vegetables

asparagus, beets, broccoli, Brussels
sprouts, cabbage, carrots, cauliflower,
celery, green beans, green leafies, kale,
mushrooms, okra, onions, snow peas,
summer squash, tomatoes and zucchini

Generally one serving of simple carbohydrate is obtained from 1/2 cup cooked vegetables or 1 cup raw vegetable or juice.

◡ COMPLEX CARBOHYDRATES ◡
GRAINS AND STARCHY VEGETABLES

Grains

The following amounts provide one serving of complex carbohydrate:

barley . . . . 1/2 cup cooked
bread . . . . 1 slice
bulgur. . . . . 1/2 cup cooked
cereals . . . . 1 ounce
   (usually 1/4 cup of a concentrated cereal such as
   grape-nuts or granola, 1/2 to 3/4 cup of flaked
   cereals and 1 cup of puffed cereals)
crackers 5
crispbread 2
grits . . . . 1/2 cup cooked
kasha . . . . 1/2 cup cooked
millet . . . . 1/2 cup cooked
oats. . . . . 1/3 cup uncooked
pasta. . . . . 1/2 cup cooked
rice (brown and wild) . . . . 1/2 cup cooked
tortillas (flour or corn) 1
wheat germ . . . . 1/4 cup

Starchy Vegetables

black-eyed peas, corn, green peas, lima
beans, parsnips, potatoes (white and sweet),
rutabagas, turnips and winter squash

Generally one serving of complex carbohydrate is obtained from 1/2 cup cooked starchy vegetable.

⌇ IDEAL PROTEIN SOURCES ∾

Serving to equal 1 ounce of protein

- nonfat milk or nonfat plain yogurt . . . . . . 4 ounces
- low-fat cheeses . . . . 1 ounce
  (less than 5 grams of fat per ounce)
  farmer's, Laughing Cow reduced-calorie
  wedges, light or fat-free cream cheese, part-skim
  mozzarella, string cheese, Jarlsberg Lite,
  Weight Watchers', Kraft Light Naturals
- 1 percent low-fat or nonfat cottage cheese
  or part-skim or fat-free ricotta . . . . 1/4 cup
- eggs (particularly use the egg whites) 1
- fish . . . . 1 ounce or
  1/4 cup flaked
- seafood (crab, lobster) . . . . 1/4 cup
- seafood (clams, shrimp, oysters, scallops). . . 5
- turkey, Cornish hens . . . . 1 ounce or 1/4
  cup chopped
- chicken . . . . 1 ounce or 1/4
  (generally, 1 cooked leg = 1 ounce protein; cup chopped
  1 cooked thigh = 1-1/2 ounces protein;
  1 cooked split breast = 2 ounces protein)

- beef, pork, lamb, veal (lean, trimmed) . . . . 1 ounce
- legumes . . . . 1/4 cup of
  black beans, garbanzo beans, Great   cooked beans
  Northern beans, kidney beans, lentils,   or 2 tablespoons
  natural peanut butter, navy beans,   of peanut
  peanuts, red beans, split peas, soybeans   butter give
  and soy products such as tofu and soy milk   approximately 1
  (*Note: Although a plant food,*   ounce of protein
  legumes contain valuable protein
  if eaten with a grain — corn, wheat,
  rice, oats — or a seed — pumpkin,
  sunflower, sesame.)

Action Step 4: Compare your food diary to the following guides to good eating. Keep in mind that these are guides for minimum portions and proper balance to achieve your desired goals for healthy living. Portion sizes may need to be increased to meet your individual body needs. Get started with these amounts for two weeks to allow your body to stabilize and then make needed adjustments.

Notice that the sample diary on page 71 and the blank diary that follows provide spaces for your protein, complex carbohydrate, simple carbohydrate and added fat. Be sure to include the time you eat, how you feel and your exercise.

For a copy of the food diary that you can reproduce, write to me at the address on page 222.

Invest the next fourteen days in making your eating style become a new, healthy lifestyle.

↭ GUIDE TO GOOD EATING ↬
WEIGHT-LOSS MEAL PLAN FOR WOMEN

Breakfast (within 1/2 hour of arising)

Complex Carbohydrate . . 1 slice whole wheat bread
OR 1/2 whole wheat English muffin
OR 3/4 cup cereal with raw bran added
(begin with 1 teaspoon bran,
gradually increasing to 2 tablespoons)

Protein . . . . 1 ounce part-skim cheese
OR 1/2 cup nonfat plain yogurt
OR 3/4 cup skim milk for cereal
OR 1 egg (limit whole eggs to 3 times
per week) or 1/4 cup egg substitute

Simple Carbohydrate . . . 1 small piece fresh fruit

Morning Snack

Carbohydrate . . . . 3 whole grain crackers
OR 1 small piece fresh fruit
OR 1 rice cake or Wasa bread

Protein . . . . 1 ounce part-skim cheese or lean meat
OR 1/2 cup nonfat plain yogurt with
1 teaspoon all-fruit jam

Lunch

Complex Carbohydrate . . 2 slices whole wheat bread
OR 1 baked potato
OR 1 whole wheat pita bread

Protein . . . . 2 ounces part-skim cheese
OR 2 ounces cooked poultry, fish or
lean roast beef
OR 1/2 cup cooked legumes

Simple Carbohydrate . . . 1 small piece fresh fruit
OR 1 cup noncreamed soup

Healthy Munchie . . . . . raw vegetable salad with no-oil
(optional)   salad dressing

Added Fat (optional) . . . . 1 teaspoon mayonnaise (or
1 tablespoon light mayonnaise)
OR 1 teaspoon butter or margarine
OR 1 teaspoon olive oil or canola oil
OR 1 tablespoon salad dressing

Afternoon Snack

Repeat earlier snack choices.

Dinner

Complex Carbohydrate . . 1/2 cup rice or pasta
OR 1/2 cup starchy vegetable

Protein . . . . 2 to 3 ounces cooked chicken, turkey,
fish, seafood or lean roast beef
OR 1/2 cup cooked legumes

Simple Carbohydrate . . . 1 cup nonstarchy vegetable
OR 1 small piece fresh fruit

Healthy Munchie . . . . . raw vegetable salad with no-oil
(optional)   salad dressing

Added Fat (optional) . . . 1 teaspoon butter or margarine
OR 1 teaspoon olive oil
OR 1 tablespoon salad dressing

Evening Snack

1 small piece fresh fruit OR 3 cups microwave light popcorn

Free Items

raw vegetables, mustard, vinegar, lemon juice, no-oil salad dressing

◟ GUIDE TO GOOD EATING ◞
WEIGHT-MAINTENANCE MEAL PLAN FOR WOMEN AND WEIGHT-LOSS MEAL PLAN FOR MEN

Breakfast (within 1/2 hour of arising)

Complex Carbohydrate . . 2 slices whole wheat bread
OR 1 whole wheat English muffin
OR 1-1/2 cups cereal with raw bran
added (begin with 1 teaspoon bran,
gradually increasing to 2 tablespoons)

Protein . . . . 2 ounces part-skim cheese
OR 1 cup skim milk for cereal
OR 2 eggs (limit whole eggs to 2 times
per week) or 1/2 cup egg substitute

Simple Carbohydrate . . . 1 piece fresh fruit

Morning Snack

Carbohydrate . . . . 5 whole grain crackers
OR 1 piece fresh fruit
OR 2 rice cakes or Wasa breads

Protein . . . . 2 ounces part-skim cheese or lean meat
OR 2 tablespoons natural peanut
butter (limit peanut butter to one
time per day)
OR 1 cup nonfat plain yogurt with
1 teaspoon all-fruit jam

Lunch

Complex Carbohydrate . . 2 slices whole wheat bread
OR 1 baked potato
OR 1 whole wheat pita bread

Protein . . . . 3 ounces part-skim cheese
OR 3 ounces cooked poultry,
fish or lean roast beef
OR 3/4 cup cooked legumes

Simple Carbohydrate . . . 1 piece fresh fruit
OR 1 cup noncreamed soup

Healthy Munchie . . . . . raw vegetable salad with no-oil
(optional)   salad dressing

Added Fat (optional) . . . 1 teaspoon mayonnaise (or
                            1 tablespoon light mayonnaise)
                            OR 1 teaspoon butter or margarine
                            OR 1 teaspoon olive oil or canola oil
                            OR 1 tablespoon salad dressing

Afternoon Snack

Repeat earlier snack choices
OR 1/2 cup trail mix (recipe on page 54).

Dinner

Complex Carbohydrate . . 1 cup rice or pasta
                          OR 1 cup starchy vegetable

Protein . . . . 3 to 4 ounces cooked chicken, turkey,
                            fish, seafood or lean roast beef
                            OR 1 cup cooked legumes

Simple Carbohydrate . . . 1 cup nonstarchy vegetable
                           OR 1 piece fresh fruit

Healthy Munchie . . . . . raw vegetable salad with no-oil
(optional)   salad dressing

Added Fat (optional) . . . 1 teaspoon butter or margarine
                            OR 1 teaspoon olive oil
                            OR 2 tablespoons sour cream
                            OR 1 tablespoon salad dressing

Evening Snack

Repeat earlier snack choices
OR 3/4 cup cereal with 1/2 cup skim milk.

Free Items

raw vegetables, mustard, vinegar, lemon juice, no-oil salad dressing

࿂ GUIDE TO GOOD EATING ࿂
WEIGHT-MAINTENANCE MEAL PLAN FOR MEN

Breakfast (within 1/2 hour of arising)

Complex Carbohydrate . . 2 slices whole wheat bread
OR 1 whole wheat English muffin
OR 1-1/2 cups cereal with raw bran
added (begin with 1 teaspoon bran,
gradually increasing to 2 tablespoons)

Protein . . . . 2 ounces part-skim cheese
OR 2 tablespoons natural peanut
butter (limit to one time per day)
OR 1 cup skim milk for cereal
OR 2 eggs (limit whole eggs to 2 times
per week) or 1/2 cup egg substitute

Simple Carbohydrate . . . 1 piece fresh fruit

Morning Snack

Carbohydrate . . . . 5 whole grain crackers
OR 2 rice cakes or Wasa breads
AND 1 piece fresh fruit

Protein . . . . 2 ounces part-skim cheese or lean meat
OR 2 tablespoons natural peanut
butter (limit peanut butter to one
time per day)
OR 1 cup nonfat plain yogurt with
1 teaspoon all-fruit jam

Lunch

Complex Carbohydrate . . 2 slices whole wheat bread
OR 1 baked potato
OR 1 whole wheat pita bread

Protein . . . . 4 ounces part-skim cheese
OR 4 ounces cooked poultry,
fish or lean roast beef
OR 1 cup cooked legumes

Simple Carbohydrate . . . 1 piece fresh fruit
AND 1 cup noncreamed soup

Healthy Munchie . . . . .   raw vegetable salad with no-oil
(optional)   salad dressing

Added Fat (optional) . . . 1 teaspoon mayonnaise (or
                                       1 tablespoon light mayonnaise)
                                    OR 1 teaspoon butter or margarine
                                    OR 1 teaspoon olive oil or canola oil
                                    OR 1 tablespoon salad dressing

Afternoon Snack

Repeat earlier snack choices
OR 1/2 cup trail mix (recipe on page 54).

Dinner

Complex Carbohydrate . . 1-1/2 cups rice or pasta
                                     OR 1-1/2 cups starchy vegetable

Protein . . . .   4 ounces cooked chicken, turkey,
                                        fish, seafood or lean roast beef
                                    OR 1 cup cooked legumes

Simple Carbohydrate . . . 1 cup nonstarchy vegetable
                                    AND 1 piece fresh fruit

Healthy Munchie . . . . .   raw vegetable salad with no-oil
(optional)   salad dressing

Added Fat (optional) . . . 1 teaspoon butter or margarine
                                    OR 1 teaspoon olive oil or canola oil
                                    OR 2 tablespoons sour cream
                                    OR 1 tablespoon salad dressing

Evening Snack

Repeat earlier snack choices OR any power snack (see pages 51 and
52) OR 1 cup cereal with 1 cup skim milk.

Free Items

raw vegetables, mustard, vinegar, lemon juice, no-oil salad dressing

~: FOOD DIARY :~

Your Name *Patti Martin*_____ Week Beginning *August 29*_____

Day	Breakfast	Lunch	Dinner	Comments & Exercise
MONDAY	Protein: 6:35 *2 eggs* Complex Carb: *2 slices toast* Simple Carb: *1 pc. fruit* Added Fat: Snack: 10:00 *c: 6 crackers* *p: 1 string cheese*	Protein: 11:45 *1 chicken breast* Complex Carb: *1 lg. baked potato* Simple Carb: *1 side vegetable* Added Fat: *1 tbsp. sour cream* Snack: 2:30 *1/2 turkey* *sandwich*	Protein: 6:45 *salmon steak* Complex Carb: *wild rice* Simple Carb: *broccoli* *mixed green salad* Added Fat: *salad dressing* Snack: 9:20 *cereal and milk*	*up at 6:30 - 6 oz.* *apple juice; walked* *40 minutes* *3:00 - getting* *tired* *3:45 - feel better* *after snack* *9:20 - not* *hungry; still* *had snack*
TUESDAY	Protein: Complex Carb: Simple Carb: Added Fat: Snack:	Protein: Complex Carb: Simple Carb: Added Fat: Snack:	Protein: Complex Carb: Simple Carb: Added Fat: Snack:	
WEDNESDAY	Protein: Complex Carb: Simple Carb: Added Fat: Snack:	Protein: Complex Carb: Simple Carb: Added Fat: Snack:	Protein: Complex Carb: Simple Carb: Added Fat: Snack:	

Action Step 4: Sample

↙ FOOD DIARY ↝

Your Name _____ Week Beginning _____

Day	Breakfast	Lunch	Dinner	Comments & Exercise
MONDAY	Protein:	Protein:	Protein:	
	Complex Carb:	Complex Carb:	Complex Carb:	
	Simple Carb:	Simple Carb:	Simple Carb:	
	Added Fat:	Added Fat:	Added Fat:	
	Snack:	Snack:	Snack:	
TUESDAY	Protein:	Protein:	Protein:	
	Complex Carb:	Complex Carb:	Complex Carb:	
	Simple Carb:	Simple Carb:	Simple Carb:	
	Added Fat:	Added Fat:	Added Fat:	
	Snack:	Snack:	Snack:	
WEDNESDAY	Protein:	Protein:	Protein:	
	Complex Carb:	Complex Carb:	Complex Carb:	
	Simple Carb:	Simple Carb:	Simple Carb:	
	Added Fat:	Added Fat:	Added Fat:	
	Snack:	Snack:	Snack:	

Day	Breakfast	Lunch	Dinner	Comments & Exercise
THURSDAY	Protein: Complex Carb: Simple Carb: Added Fat: Snack:	Protein: Complex Carb: Simple Carb: Added Fat: Snack:	Protein: Complex Carb: Simple Carb: Added Fat: Snack:	
FRIDAY	Protein: Complex Carb: Simple Carb: Added Fat: Snack:	Protein: Complex Carb: Simple Carb: Added Fat: Snack:	Protein: Complex Carb: Simple Carb: Added Fat: Snack:	
SATURDAY	Protein: Complex Carb: Simple Carb: Added Fat: Snack:	Protein: Complex Carb: Simple Carb: Added Fat: Snack:	Protein: Complex Carb: Simple Carb: Added Fat: Snack:	
SUNDAY	Protein: Complex Carb: Simple Carb: Added Fat: Snack:	Protein: Complex Carb: Simple Carb: Added Fat: Snack:	Protein: Complex Carb: Simple Carb: Added Fat: Snack:	

↝ Eat Lean ↜

Fat-free cookies...fat-free cupcakes...fat-free frozen yogurt — the grocery shelves scream with new products engineered to be free of fat. The words *light* and *low-fat* on labels are being replaced with the new buzz word of health — *fat-free.*

These days it's hard to pick up a magazine or newspaper without reading something about cutting out the fat from our diets. But the truth is that we can get overwhelmed with the task and frustrations abound because not much information is available on how to accomplish it.

The common questions I hear are: How do I identify and cut out fatty foods? What can I eat? I've grown up in a world where food's flavor was found in seasoning with fats. How can I ever enjoy foods cooked dry and plain? Or, I closed my kitchen a few years back, and we eat out most of the time. Is there any way to eat well when eating out?

As I hear these pleas for help day after day, I become convinced that the story about fat has become a version of "The Good, the Bad...and the Very Confusing!"

Fortunately, you need not cut out all traces of fat in your diet. Actually, too little fat in your diet can be as undesirable as too much fat; it is necessary for human life! But a little fat goes a long way; we require only small amounts of fat from foods each day. When fat-laden foods are eaten to excess, the body has no choice but to store the fat, either on the body or in the bloodstream. This bad news has made fat the nutritional bad guy of the nineties. The most up-to-date research continues to point to fat as a primary culprit in obesity and disease.[1]

Fat Makes Us Fat

The excess fat calories we consume are converted and stored as fat more readily than those from other sources. Fat is a more concentrated source of calories (all fats contain twice as many calories as equal amounts of carbohydrate or proteins, about 9 calories per gram, or 120 calories per tablespoon). In addition, the body is more efficient in storing fat as fat. In other words, 100 calories of butter (one tablespoon) are more likely to go to your hips than 100 calories of whole wheat bread (about two slices).

This is why the weight control experts of today consider trimming the fat from our diets to be much more important in weight loss than just watching calories.

Of course, fatness or thinness is not the only issue involved in our food choices. Even if you have been blessed with a metabolism that burns brightly, allowing you to maintain your weight easily, don't believe you can eat all the fatty foods you want. You may not be seeing the problem on a scale or on your waistline, but excess fat intake can bring problems nonetheless.

Consider these vital facts about fat and your health:

- Excess fat intake increases cholesterol levels and your risk of heart disease and stroke. While research shows that saturated fat is the main culprit, it also shows that any type of fat can cause problems.

- Excess fat intake increases risk of cancer, particularly of the colon and breast. Fat alone is presently implicated in one-third of all cancer deaths.[2]

- Excess fat intake increases risk of gallbladder disease.

- Excess fat intake, particularly saturated fat, elevates blood pressure, regardless of weight.

- Excess fat fed to animals with a genetic susceptibility to diabetes has made them more likely to develop the disease. People with a family history of diabetes can cut the percentage of fat in their diets as one step of prevention of this disease.

- And, again, it's fat that makes us fat!

It's no wonder that Leviticus 3:17 warns: "This is a lasting ordinance for the generations to come, wherever you live: You must not eat any fat...."

If your cholesterol count is normal, your blood pressure low and your family tree free of cancer, heart disease and diabetes, these facts may seem irrelevant to you. Being free from all risk factors is rare but is a blessing that can be enhanced with a healthy way of eating. Preventing the diseases of tomorrow is great, but the reason to change is for *today!*

The daily eating of low-fat proteins, whole grains, fruits and vegetables gives us higher levels of energy and alertness, better stress management and even improved memory and sleep.

These facts point to a less-is-more lifestyle choice: *Less* fat in our diets means *more* wellness and protection from disease and weight struggles. But entering this low-fat lifestyle can be tricky. It is estimated that today's American takes in approximately 40 percent of his daily calories from fat. Chances are you may be eating more than you realize.

A day's intake of sixty grams of fat may sound like a lot — until you realize that's the fat content of a fast-food taco salad. Actually, the typical adult eats the fat equivalent of one stick of butter a day!

How Much Is Enough?

It is recommended that you limit your dietary fat intake to 25 to 30 percent of total calorie limit. Moderately active women need approximately 2,000 calories daily for maintaining weight; moderately active men need about 2,500 calories. For weight loss goals, 1,200 calories are a good day's limit for women; 1,500 calories for men. To determine the 25 percent fat allowance, use this formula:

25 percent x 1,200 calories = 300 calories

300 calories divided by 9 calories per gram of fat = 33 grams maximum fat suggested each day

According to the formula, the number of fat grams recommended for your daily calorie limit would be as follows:

Daily Calories	Suggested Fat Grams
1,200 calories	33 grams
1,500 calories	42 grams
1,800 calories	50 grams
2,000 calories	55 grams
2,500 calories	67 grams

Like any worthy goal, reducing our personal fat intake requires some effort and commitment — to learn new ways to season foods without fat, to order more healthfully at restaurants and to discover positive snack foods. But the benefits far exceed the effort. Smart eating does not doom you to nutritional martyrdom and eating foods that taste like cardboard. Nor do you have to become a chemical analyst to stay within these guidelines while dining out, grocery shopping or cooking. Everyday foods are full of potent healing ingredients that boost energy and help you feel and look better. With the creativity and innovation available today, tasty foods that are good for you are popping up everywhere!

The first line of defense in fighting any battle is to identify your enemies. In the war against excess fat, the enemy's hideouts are meats, poultry, dairy products and nuts, along with butter and oil toppings such as salad dressings and mayonnaise.

Cutting fat is nearly impossible for the long-term without adding in fiber. Because fat in food leaves you feeling satisfied when you've eaten, you need to create that same feeling of fullness without the fat by increasing the amount of fiber in your meals. Grains, fruits and vegetables are excellent sources of fill-you-up nutrition and are low in fat — provided they aren't drowned in butter or sauces.

I was raised on fried chicken, mashed potatoes with gravy and green beans cooked in bacon grease. Maybe you were too. Embracing a lifestyle of better eating and better living meant a lot more to me than cutting out candy bars. It meant finding ways to enjoy flavorful foods — without the grease. Believing that the experience of eating was meant to be a pleasurable one, there was no way I was going to accept a life filled with dry, tasteless food. I had to establish new ways of shopping, cooking and dining out. Let me encourage you to do the same.

Because good health starts at mealtime, use this guide to help you lighten your diet one step at a time:

✌ Trim the Fat When Cooking ⌇

- Eat more fish and skinless poultry and fewer red meats. If you eat red meats, buy lean cuts and trim well (before and after cooking), cooking them in a way that diminishes fat, such as grilling, broiling or roasting on a rack.

- Use marinades, flavored vinegars, plain yogurt or juices when grilling or broiling to tenderize leaner cuts of meat and seal in their moisture and flavor. Mix these marinades with fresh or dried herbs such as basil, oregano and parsley to add flavors.

- Limit protein portions to five ounces precooked. After cooking, the size will be that of a deck of cards. This is the typical lunch portion of fish or chicken served in a restaurant. The typical dinner portion is nine ounces, great for sharing or halving for a "doggie bag."

- Let rice, pasta, potatoes and vegetables become the centerpiece of your meals.

- Use nonstick cooking sprays and skillets to brown meats without grease, and sauté ingredients in stocks and broths rather than fats and oils. If a recipe calls for basting in butter or the meat's own juices, baste instead with tomato or lemon juice or stocks.

- Skim the fat from soups, stocks and meat drippings. Refrigerate and remove the hardened surface layer of fat before reheating. As you do, think about that fat hardening in your body and how you are doing yourself a great favor.

- Use legumes (dried beans and peas) as a main dish. These meat substitutes make a high nutrition, low-fat meal; try them at least twice each week. If beans have been gas-producing in the past, try Beano (available from your pharmacy); it's a natural enzyme that works wonders for digesting beans and other gas-forming foods while your body is becoming more tolerant on its own.

- Substitute plain, nonfat yogurt or fat-free ricotta cheese in dips or sauces calling for sour cream or mayonnaise. Also use these as toppings for baked potatoes and chili. (And don't forget low-fat, flavorful salsa, a hot topping for anything!)

- Use two egg whites or 1/4 cup egg substitute in place of one whole egg. Egg whites are pure protein; egg yolks are pure fat and cholesterol!

- Rarely, if ever, eat animal organ meats, such as liver, sweetbreads or brains. They are loaded with fats and cholesterol.

ᴠᴗ Trim the Fat When Grocery Shopping ᴖ

- Switch from whole-milk dairy products to skim or 1 percent milk, buttermilk or nonfat plain yogurt. Look for fat-free or lower-fat versions of favorite cheeses such as ricotta, pot or farmer's, skim-milk mozzarella, cottage cheese and fat-free or light cream cheese. Check the label to be sure they have fewer than five grams of fat per ounce.

  But beware of nondairy products touting themselves as fat-free. You need to ask yourself the question, If it's a fat (mayonnaise, salad dressing, margarine, ice cream), and it's made to be fat-free, what is it? Often the product is a witch's brew of chemicals, thickeners and dyes manufactured to feel and taste like fat in the mouth. Exceptions are some of the fat-free dairy products, such as fat-free cheeses, yogurts and the like. They are made from skim milk, generally with little or no additives.

Also beware of products with hydrogenated oil listed as one of the first three ingredients; it is a fat that has been chemically saturated by manufacturers.

- At the deli, go for the leanest cuts. Select sliced turkey or chicken, lean ham and low-fat cheeses instead of the usual luncheon meats. Limit use of high-fat, high-sodium sausages and processed meats, hot dogs, bacon and salami.

- Use this formula for figuring fat percentage of calories when assessing whether new food products are as good as they claim:

9 calories per gram of fat × grams of fat ÷ calories per serving = % of calories from fat

Example: A food giving 100 calories per one-ounce serving contains 9 grams of fat. So the equation would look like this:

9 grams of fat × 9 calories per gram = 81 calories ÷ 100 total calories = 81% of calories from fat (way too much!)

Buy foods that contain less than 25 percent of their calories from fat. If a hundred-calorie serving contains more than three grams of fat, it's too much.

- Buy whole grain and freshly baked breads and rolls. They have more flavor and do not need butter or margarine to taste good.

- Use the new all-fruit jams on breads or toast, rather than fat spreads like butter or margarine.

- Keep an abundant supply of fresh fruits and precut, munchy vegetables on hand for snacking. Buy light popcorn, breads and low-fat crackers rather than chips and cookies. Substitute sorbet or frozen juice bars for ice cream. Nonfat frozen yogurts may also be used sparingly; although they contain no fat, they are higher in sugar than ice cream.

༄ Trim the Fat When Dining Out ༄

- Choose a restaurant that you know and trust for quality. When you have control over where you are dining, plan ahead for restaurants with a willingness to prepare foods in a healthy way upon request. Many progressive and responsible restaurants now offer healthful menu selections.

- Order fats on the side in restaurant meals, and apply them in limited quantities. The typical restaurant meal contains the fat equivalent of twelve to fourteen pats of butter in the sauces, dressings, toppings and spreads.

- Make special requests. It's your health, your money and your waistline. Most foods can be prepared without fat and butter; just order meats, poultry or fish grilled without fat, and sauces on the side. Ask for fresh vegetables steamed without added butter.

- Watch the portions. The typical plate gives you twice as much as you need. Believe me, there are no rewards for cleaning your plate! You have other choices: Order an appetizer instead of an entree, or order a lunch portion at dinner; share one meal with a willing partner, or take leftovers home for a great meal tomorrow.

Think of a move toward nutritious, low-fat eating as a permanent change instead of a dieting regime. Don't keep a calculator at your bedside, and don't get stuck in a deprivation mode. Be easy on yourself and go slowly, taking practical, feasible steps one at a time. Focus on good foods, well-prepared, and your desires will shift. Give your tastebuds time to return to how they were created. High-fat foods will have less and less appeal as you eat foods that give you energy, better digestion and a sense of well-being.

Action Step 5: Keep a new diary of eating for three days and evaluate it for "grease traps." Replace them with lower-fat versions. Notice the sample on the next page for ways to cut fat.

✧ FOOD DIARY ✧

Your Name _Patti Martin_ _____ Week Beginning _September 3_ _____

Day	Breakfast	Lunch	Dinner	Comments & Exercise
MONDAY	Time: 6:30 _Nutri Grain cereal with_ ~~_2% 1%_~~ _1% milk_ _banana_ _water_	Time: 12:45 ~~_Taco Salad_~~ _2 soft tacos_ _water_	Time: 6:15 ~~_Fettucine Alfredo_~~ _Fettucine with marinara sauce_ _water_	_feel great!_ _more energy_
	~~_peanut butter crackers_~~ _string cheese + Harvest Crisp_	~~_microwave popcorn_~~ _light popcorn_	~~_ice cream_~~ _cereal w/milk_	
TUESDAY	Time:	Time:	Time:	
	Snack:	Snack:	Snack:	
WEDNESDAY	Time:	Time:	Time:	
	Snack:	Snack:	Snack:	

Action Step 5: Sample

SEVEN

WATER IS
THE BEVERAGE
OF CHAMPIONS

THE SIGN BY my sink said it all: *"Remember: Water Is Our Most Valuable Resource."* The city of San Francisco was using the sign to entreat hotel guests like me to use water wisely and *sparingly*. I was struck with the irony that I encourage people to use water wisely and *abundantly*.

With the body being comprised primarily of water (water is 92 percent of our blood plasma, 80 percent of our muscle mass, 60 percent of our red blood cells and 50 percent of everything else in our bodies), water is an important ingredient to good health.

Most Americans, however, have grown up drinking just about anything but water. We list our favorite beverages as soda, coffee, tea, juice, Kool-aid — with water being good only for swallowing pills, washing away dirt and brushing our teeth. Although we often hear that we should drink water, it's easier to reach for something else. And we pay a price. We miss out on water's benefits.

Water is an essential nutrient. Without food a person can survive (although not well!) for days, even months. But without water the human body can survive only three to five days. It is critical for maintaining proper fluid balance. Along with proper protein and salt intake, water works to release excess stores of fluid, much like priming a pump. It is *the* natural diuretic; no other beverage works like water.

Water is the only liquid we consume that doesn't require the body to work to metabolize or excrete it. Even juices do not provide the solid benefits of pure, wonderful water, since they require our bodies to process the substances they contain. With soft drinks, our bodies have to work overtime to process and excrete the chemicals and colorings.

Many other beverages, particularly those containing caffeine, actually remove more water than contained in the beverage itself. Furthermore, coffee, tea and some sodas contain tannic acid, a product that interferes with iron and calcium absorption and competes for excretion with other bodily waste products such as uric acid. When not properly excreted, this uric acid can build up in the body and crystallize around the joints. This buildup leads to joint pain in elbows, shoulders, knees and feet, especially former injury spots, and is a sort of gouty arthritis. Men are particulary prone to uric acid excesses. This is one reason why a glass of tea or coffee — although fluid-based — just doesn't do the job.

Being a mild laxative, water allows proper bowel function and waste elimination. It actually activates the fiber you eat, allowing it to pass through the gastrointestinal tract easily and quickly. Without proper water, fiber becomes a difficult-to-pass glue in your colon.

Water is also valuable for maintaining proper muscle tone. It allows muscles to contract naturally, which prevents dehydration.

Proper hydration is a crucial part of a winning strategy for professional or amateur athletes. When dehydrated, the muscles are more injury-prone and will not work to optimum performance. When not receiving proper water, the muscles will only work to 35 percent of their capability.

One last merit (for the age-conscious): Water works to keep the skin healthy and resilient. It can honestly be labeled an anti-aging ingredient!

Although you may drink other beverages, do not let them become a substitute for the beverage your body likes best — the beverage of champions.

How Much Do I Need?

My answer is always the same: eight to ten glasses each day; more if you drink coffees, teas or sodas; and much more when you exercise. My response usually brings cries of anguish. But as you begin to meet this need by drinking more water, your natural thirst will increase. You may find that drinking water is habit-forming; the more you drink, the more you want.

Start increasing your intake any way you can — through a straw, in a sports sipper, from a silver pitcher. Just drink it!

Try filling a two-quart container with water each morning, then make sure it's all gone before you go to bed. I also encourage a habit of drinking an eight-ounce glass of water right after each meal and snack through the day. If you are eating as often as you should — every two and one-half to three hours — this will provide a large portion of the fluid you need each day.

Purified or bottled water is a nice treat, and any glass of water is refreshing with lemon or lime slices added.

When More Is Better

You will need more water when you are exercising and even more when you travel, especially if you fly.

A dry airplane cabin is ten times more arid than the Sahara

Desert, causing you to lose fluids through your skin. This condition can easily lead to dehydration, with the results of puffy hands and ankles and a generally bloated feeling. The key for preventing this is to drink eight to twelve ounces of replacement fluids each hour you are in the air. The best fluids: water, sparkling water or club soda, and fruit juices. The worst: caffeinated drinks (coffees, teas and sodas) and alcoholic beverages; they intensify the dehydration.

Any type of exercise, particularly when strenuous, greatly increases your need for replacement fluids.

Adults and children alike should drink plenty of water before, during and after exercise — approximately six ounces every twenty minutes.

Beware of fluid-replacement sports drinks. They are generally too high in certain electrolytes (sodium and potassium) and sugars and are not as good a choice as cool, clear water. If you drink them, they should be diluted three parts water to one part sports drink.

Is Tap Water OK?

If you drink tap water, the taste may improve after refrigerating it for twenty-four hours (the chlorine, added to disinfect community drinking water, will dissipate). This can be an inexpensive way to get the more refreshing taste of bottled water without the cost.

Be sure not to let the bottled versus tap versus treated water controversy get in the way of your health. Public water systems today are well monitored for safety; bottled water companies are just now beginning to fall under similar standards. Your choice of which water to drink comes down to taste, cost and availability, but don't miss out on it.

As the sign said, "Water is our most valuable resource" — at least for the physical body!

A Word About Caffeine

A relatively mild stimulant, caffeine is among the world's most widely used and addictive drugs. Ironically, caffeine remains an acceptable way of artificially stimulating the brain at a time when society is being exhorted to "just say no." Caffeine works by blocking one of the brain's natural sedatives, a chemical called adenosine. It stimulates the central nervous system and can elevate moods. A single cup of coffee can seem to work energy miracles when needed.

Like other drugs, however, there is a downside to caffeine; too much causes a surge of adrenaline. But when the spurt is over, power levels plummet. Even small amounts of it may cause side effects, including restlessness and disturbed sleep, heart palpitations, stomach irritation, fibrocystic breast disease and diarrhea. It can promote irritability, anxiety and mood disturbances. Caffeine can also aggravate premenstrual syndrome in women.

The stimulant effect is thought to kick in with consumption of some 150 to 250 milligrams of caffeine — the amount in one to two cups of brewed coffee or three glasses of iced tea. And because caffeine is also found in soda (regular and diet), chocolate and even decongestant cold pills, it adds up quickly.

Do you need to cut out caffeine altogether? Not necessarily. I do encourage you, however, to cut back slowly to this ceiling of 250 milligrams. And if, after cutting back to this amount, you still experience any of the above-mentioned side effects of caffeine, I would suggest withdrawing altogether.

Withdrawal is the word for cutting back on caffeine consumption, and that is why you must do so gradually. Many people experience zombie-like fatigue and headaches from caffeine withdrawal, and the symptoms may last for up to five days. Eating small, balanced meals throughout the day will stabilize the body chemistries and reduce the reliance on caffeine for energy. Nonetheless, set a goal and cut back slowly. If you focus on drinking more water than you have in the past, you won't have room for the other beverages!

> **Action Step 6:** Review your eating (and drinking!) pattern for the last three days. How much water have you been drinking compared to how much your body needs?

EIGHT

VARIETY
IS THE
SPICE OF LIFE

THE BEAUTIFUL THING about good, balanced nutrition is this: Everything fits together in such a perfect way that just focusing on eating (early, often, balanced and lean) will give you a blessing of essential nutrients. You don't have to analyze your intake continually to be sure you've had your zinc today.

What you are responsible to do is to choose healthy foods with a sense of balance and variety — the cornerstones of good nutrition.

Your health doesn't depend on a single food or a single meal. No one food is perfect; no one food contains all the nutrients you need.

Healthy variety occurs when you make good food choices over a period of time.

Be sure to provide whole grain, low-fat meals that are full of a variety of brightly colored fruits and vegetables. The bright coloring is a sign of the nutritional content of a vegetable or fruit; generally the more vivid the coloring, the more essential nutrients it holds. That deep orange or red coloring in carrots, sweet potatoes, cantaloupes, apricots, peaches and strawberries signals their vitamin A content. Dark green leafy vegetables such as turnip or mustard greens, spinach, romaine lettuce, Brussels sprouts and broccoli are loaded with vitamin A as well as folic acid. Vitamin C is found in more than just citrus; it is also power-packed into strawberries, cantaloupes, tomatoes, green peppers and broccoli. Remember: You may not be able to tell a book by its cover, but you can tell the power of a fruit or veggie by its color!

Are you still saying yuck to the same veggies you didn't like when you were young? Open your mind, your taste buds, your likes and dislikes, your schedule and your menu to these storehouses of nutritional power — they are worth it.

Breaking the Rut

Healthy eating doesn't need to be anything less than enjoyable, tasty and full of variety. Yet for many people, healthy eating means eating in a rut, a boring rut.

We settle into a limited variety of dishes with which we feel safe and don't have to think about much. We don't want to have to make decisions; it's just easier to have the same bowl of cereal for breakfast, a "ditto" turkey sandwich at lunch and a piece of baked chicken for dinner.

Why such a rut? It's easier for us to trust the rut than to trust ourselves to make healthy choices. Some people are subconsciously trying to work wonders, thinking that just the right (or only one) combination of food will work and be safe. Some people seem to punish themselves with the same old, boring foods, thinking they are paying some kind of penance for their last binge. Others, who don't care enough about themselves to do anything differently, feed themselves with as much forethought and effort as they feed their pets.

So what's the problem with ruts? Time and again I see people set up to overindulge as soon as they get the taste of anything more exciting. Then once they get off track, it becomes very difficult to get back on track — since, to them, "on track" means returning to the same old, boring rut.

That's the emotional reason ruts are deadly. There are also some nutritional ones.

Eating a variety of foods in their whole form provides you with a gamut of vitamins and minerals, including as yet hidden benefits.

An example of this is what we've learned in recent years about broccoli. Research shows that the very substance that makes broccoli, broccoli — or cauliflower, cauliflower — has cancer-preventive properties. This flavoring substance is found only in the cruciferous vegetable family, such as cabbage, cauliflower, Brussels sprouts and broccoli. If you don't eat these vegetables, you don't get the benefit of their protective action against this deadly disease.

And there are countless more stories of protection-through-food pouring out of the scientific literature today. A report published in 1993 in the *Journal of Nutrition and Cancer* cited that 128 out of 156 studies reviewed showed a clear link between disease protection and a variety of fruits and vegetables.

Try some of the meal ideas and recipes that follow to get free of your eating rut and to enjoy a whole new world of food. Each recipe is followed by the serving size to meet minimum (weight) needs. The Guides to Good Eating on page 65 through page 70 will give you more direction about the serving sizes to meet your particular needs.

∽ RECIPES ∾

✌ BREAKFAST ON THE GO ✌

Quick, Easy and Delicious!

Orange Vanilla French Toast

4 egg whites, lightly beaten
1/2 cup skim milk
2 tablespoons frozen,
   unsweetened orange juice
   concentrate, undiluted
1 teaspoon vanilla

1/2 teaspoon ground
   cinnamon
4 slices whole wheat bread
4 tablespoons all-fruit jam
nonstick cooking spray

Beat together the egg whites, milk, orange juice concentrate, vanilla and cinnamon. Add the bread slices one at a time, letting the bread absorb the liquid; this may take a few minutes. Coat a skillet with nonstick cooking spray and heat. Gently lift each bread slice with a spatula and place it in the skillet; cook on each side until golden brown.

Serve each slice of toast topped with 1 tablespoon all-fruit jam. Freeze the leftovers in individual freezer bags. When ready to use a slice, toast it to thaw and heat.

Makes 4 servings, each giving 1 complex carbohydrate (the bread), 1 ounce protein (the egg whites and milk) and 1 simple carbohydrate (the juice and the all-fruit jam).

Nutritional Profile per Serving
28 g carbohydrate; 8 g protein; 1.5 g fat; 11% calories from fat;
2 mg cholesterol; 250 mg sodium; 152 calories

Shake-'em-up Shake With Bran Muffin

One serving of a muffin and a shake gives 1 complex carbohydrate (the muffin); 1 ounce protein (the milk) and 2 simple carbohydrates (the juice and the raisins).

Shake-'em-up Shake

8 ounces (1 cup) skim or 1% milk
1/2 cup fresh orange juice

1 teaspoon vanilla
4 to 5 ice cubes

Pour all of the ingredients in a large cup with a lid. Shake wildly and drink up!

Nutritional Profile per Serving
25 g carbohydrate; 9 g protein; .6 g fat; 4% calories from fat; 4 mg cholesterol; 127 mg sodium; 142 calories

Spiced Bran Muffins

1/4 cup molasses
3 tablespoons honey
2 large egg whites
1/4 cup plain, nonfat yogurt
1/4 cup 1% or skim milk
1/4 cup wheat bran
1/4 cup oat bran
1 cup whole wheat pastry
  flour

1-1/2 teaspoons baking
  powder
1 teaspoon ground ginger
1 teaspoon ground cloves
1 teaspoon cinnamon
1/4 cup chopped pecans
1/4 cup golden raisins
nonstick cooking spray

Preheat oven to 350 degrees. Warm the molasses and the honey in the microwave or in a saucepan until they just begin to steam (about 110 degrees). Let the mixture cool. Whisk the egg whites, yogurt and milk together until blended. Add the molasses-honey mixture while whisking. Gently stir in the brans, the flour, the baking powder and the spices; then fold in the pecans and the raisins.

Spray a 12-cup muffin tin with nonstick spray and fill each cup two-thirds full with batter. Bake for 15 to 20 minutes or until a toothpick inserted into the center of a muffin comes out clean. Serve warm, or freeze individually in freezer bags to use later.

Nutritional Profile per Muffin
21 g carbohydrate; 3 g protein; 1.7 g fat; 15% calories from fat;
0 mg cholesterol; 28 mg sodium; 106 calories

Breakfast Sundae Supreme

1/2 banana, quartered
  lengthwise
1/2 cup nonfat ricotta cheese
1/4 cup strawberries, sliced
1/4 cup crushed pineapple,
  canned in own juice

2 tablespoons grape-nuts or
  low-fat granola
1 teaspoon honey or all-fruit
  pourable syrup

Place the banana quarters star-fashioned on a small plate. Scoop ricotta cheese onto the center points. Surround with the other fruit; then sprinkle with cereal. Drizzle with honey or all-fruit syrup.

One serving gives 1 complex carbohydrate (the cereal), 2 ounces protein (the ricotta) and 2 simple carbohydrates (the fruit).

Nutritional Profile per Serving
42 g carbohydrate; 15 g protein; 1 g fat; 4% calories from fat;
5 mg cholesterol; 111 mg sodium; 224 calories

Hot Apple Cinnamon Oatmeal

1/3 cup old-fashioned oats
3/4 cup skim milk
1/4 cup apple juice

1 tablespoon raisins
1/2 teaspoon cinnamon
1/2 teaspoon vanilla

Bring the oats, milk and apple juice to a boil. Cook for 5 minutes, stirring occasionally. Add raisins, cinnamon and vanilla. Remove the cooked oats from the heat; cover the pan and let the oats sit for 2 to 3 minutes to thicken. This recipe also cooks well in the microwave. Combine all ingredients and cook for 3 to 4 minutes on high.

Makes 1 serving, giving 1 complex carbohydrate (oats), 1 ounce protein (milk) and 2 simple carbohydrates (the juice and raisins).

Nutritional Profile per Serving
39 g carbohydrate; 11 g protein; 2 g fat; 8% calories from fat;
3 mg cholesterol; 97 mg sodium; 217 calories

Baked Breakfast Apple

1 small Golden Delicious
   apple, cored
2 tablespoons old-fashioned
   oats
1/4 teaspoon cinnamon

1 tablespoon raisins
2 tablespoons apple juice
1/2 cup nonfat ricotta
   cheese

Place the apple in a microwaveable bowl. Mix together the oats, the cinnamon and the raisins. Fill the cavity of the cored apple with the mixture. Pour the apple juice over the apple, and cover it with plastic wrap. Microwave on high for 1 minute. Turn the dish around halfway and microwave for 1 minute more. Spoon the ricotta cheese onto a plate, and top it with the apple and the heated juice mixture.

Makes 1 serving, giving 1 complex carbohydrate (the oats), 2 ounces protein (the ricotta) and 1 simple carbohydrate (the apple, the juice and the raisins).

Nutritional Profile per Serving
30 g carbohydrate; 14 g protein; 1 g fat; 6% calories from fat;
23 mg cholesterol; 100 mg sodium; 183 calories

Scrambled Eggs Burrito

1 10" flour tortilla, preferably whole wheat
1/4 teaspoon creole seasoning
2 eggs, lightly beaten, or 1/2 cup egg substitute

2 tablespoons part-skim milk cheddar cheese, grated
1/4 cup picante sauce
nonstick cooking spray
1/4 cantaloupe, sliced

Heat a nonstick pan or griddle over medium high heat. Add the tortilla to heat and soften, turning it over after 15 seconds. After 15 seconds on the second side, remove the tortilla from the pan and wrap it in foil to keep warm. Spray the pan with nonstick spray, continuing to heat. Beat together the eggs, the grated cheese and the creole seasoning. Add to the pan and scramble. Place the egg mixture on the tortilla and spoon on the picante sauce. Wrap it up burrito-style. Serve with the sliced cantaloupe.

Makes 1 serving, giving 1 complex carbohydrate (tortilla), 3 ounces protein (eggs and cheese) and 1 simple carbohydrate (cantaloupe).

Nutritional Profile per Serving
32 g carbohydrate; 13 g protein; 5 g fat; 20% calories from fat (with egg substitute); 8 mg cholesterol; 613 mg sodium; 223 calories

Southwestern Fruit Toast

2 egg whites, lightly beaten
2 tablespoons skim milk
1/2 teaspoon vanilla
1 10" flour tortilla, preferably whole wheat

nonstick cooking spray
2 tablespoons low-fat granola
1/2 cup mixed berries
1 tablespoon all-fruit syrup

Beat together the egg whites, the milk and the vanilla. Dip the tortilla into the mixture, letting it absorb the liquid for a minute or so. Coat a nonstick skillet with nonstick spray and heat.

Gently lift the tortilla with a spatula, place it in the skillet and cook until it is golden brown on each side. Sprinkle one half of the tortilla with the granola and the fruit. Fold the tortilla over omelette style and slide it onto a plate. Drizzle it with the all-fruit syrup.

Makes 1 serving, giving 2 complex carbohydrates (the tortilla and the granola), 2 ounces protein (the egg whites and the milk) and 2 simple carbohydrates (the fruit and fruit syrup).

Nutritional Profile per Serving
44 g carbohydrate; 13.5 g protein; 2 g fat; 7% calories from fat;
8 mg cholesterol; 266 mg sodium; 249 calories

Hot Oatcakes

4 egg whites
1 cup nonfat ricotta cheese
2 tablespoons canola oil
1 teaspoon vanilla
2/3 cup old-fashioned oats,
   uncooked

1/4 teaspoon salt
nonstick cooking spray
4 tablespoons all-fruit jam or
   pourable all-fruit syrup

Measure the egg whites, the cheese, the oil, the vanilla, the oats and the salt into a blender or food processor and blend for 5 to 6 seconds. Spoon 2 tablespoons of the batter into a hot skillet sprayed with nonstick spray. Turn the pancakes when bubbles appear on the surface; cook them for 1 more minute.

For 1 serving, spread 3 pancakes with 1 tablespoon all-fruit jam or syrup. Makes 12 3-inch pancakes. Freeze the leftovers in individual freezer bags. When ready to use, toast the pancakes to thaw and heat.

Makes 4 servings, each giving 1 complex carbohydrate (the pancakes), 2 ounces protein (the ricotta and the egg whites), 1 simple carbohydrate (the jam) and 1 added fat.

Nutritional Profile per Serving
25 g carbohydrate; 12 g protein; 7 g fat; 29% calories from fat;
3 mg cholesterol; 97.5 mg sodium; 211 calories

∴ LUNCH EXPRESS ∾

Don't skip that midday meal. For a lunch that will refresh, satisfy and keep your energy high, try one of these delicious and fast, complete meals.

Pita Pizzas

1 whole wheat pita, cut in half into rounds (like a saucer)
2 tablespoons spaghetti sauce

1 -1/2 ounces or 1/3 cup part-skim or nonfat mozzarella cheese, shredded
1 small apple, cut into wedges

Preheat oven to 375 degrees. Place the two pita circles on a baking sheet. Spread each one with half of the spaghetti sauce and top each with half of the cheese. Bake for 8 to 10 minutes or until cheese is bubbly. Serve with apple wedges.

Makes one serving giving 2 complex carbohydrates (the pita bread), 2 ounces protein (the cheese) and 1 simple carbohydrate (the sauce).

Nutritional Profile per Serving
37 g carbohydrate; 15 g protein; 9 g fat; 28% calories from fat; 24 mg cholesterol; 570 mg sodium; 289 calories

Swiss Stuffed Potatoes

4 baking potatoes (about 5 ounces each)
1/2 cup part-skim or nonfat ricotta cheese
1/4 teaspoon salt
1/4 teaspoon black pepper
6 ounces part-skim or 1-1/2 cups nonfat mozzarella cheese, shredded
paprika
2 cups mixed, chopped seasonal fruit

Preheat oven to 400 degrees. Wash the potatoes and bake for 1 hour until done. Or microwave potatoes by pricking and cooking on high for 8 minutes, turning and microwaving for another 8 minutes.

Once cooked, cut the potatoes in half lengthwise and scoop out most of the pulp, leaving a 1/4-inch shell. In a bowl, mash the potato pulp with the ricotta cheese, the salt and the pepper. Stir in the mozzarella cheese and spoon the mixture into the potato shells. Sprinkle with paprika.

Increase the oven temperature to broil; broil the stuffed potato shells for 3 to 5 minutes or until they are heated through and lightly browned on top. Serve each potato with 1/2 cup mixed, chopped fruit.

Makes 4 servings of 2 halves each. Each serving gives 1 complex carbohydrate (the potato), 2 ounces protein (the cheese) and 1 simple carbohydrate (the fruit).

Nutritional Profile per Serving
28 g carbohydrate; 17 g protein; 9 g fat; 24% calories from fat; 34 mg cholesterol; 513 mg sodium; 339 calories

Turkey Tortilla Roll

1 10" flour tortilla,
  preferably whole wheat
1 teaspoon Dijon-style
  mustard
2 ounces skinned turkey
  breast, fully cooked and sliced
1/2 ounce (1 tablespoon)
  part-skim milk cheddar
  cheese, grated

1/2 tomato, cut into strips
1/4 cup romaine lettuce,
  shredded
freshly ground black pepper,
  if desired
celery and carrot sticks
10 fresh strawberries or
  other fruit

Spread the tortilla with mustard. Top with the sliced turkey, the cheese, the tomato, the lettuce and the pepper, if desired. Fold in the sides of the tortilla, roll it up burrito-style and cut it in half. Serve with celery and carrot sticks and fresh fruit.

One serving gives 1 complex carbohydrate (the tortilla), 3 ounces protein (the turkey and the cheese) and 1 simple carbohydrate (the fruit).

Nutritional Profile per Serving
31 g carbohydrate; 25 g protein; 7.9 g fat; 24% calories from fat;
49 mg cholesterol; 194 mg sodium; 296 calories

Terrific Tuna Grill

2 cans (6-1/2 ounces each) solid white tuna, water-packed, drained
1/2 cup carrots, shredded
1 stalk celery, diced
1 apple, diced (1/2 cup)
2 tablespoons light mayonnaise
2 tablespoons orange juice

3 tablespoons plain, nonfat yogurt
1 teaspoon Dijon-style mustard
1/2 teaspoon creole seasoning
2 plum tomatoes, sliced
8 slices 100% whole wheat bread
nonstick cooking spray

Combine the tuna, the carrots, the celery and the apple. In a separate bowl stir together the mayonnaise, the orange juice, the yogurt, the mustard and the creole seasoning until blended. Pour the mixture over the salad, stirring to coat it. Divide the salad into 4 portions, spreading each portion onto one slice of bread. Top each with 2 slices of tomato and the other slice of bread. Spray a nonstick skillet with nonstick cooking spray and heat on medium high. Grill the sandwiches until brown.

Makes 4 servings, each giving 2 complex carbohydrates (the bread), 3 ounces protein (the tuna) and 1 simple carbohydrate (veggies and fruit).

Nutritional Profile per Serving
37 g carbohydrate; 28 g protein; 4.7 g fat; 14% calories from fat; 38 mg cholesterol; 567 mg sodium; 300 calories

Grilled Turkey and Cheese Sandwich

2 teaspoons Dijon-style
  mustard
2 slices 100% whole wheat
  bread
1 ounce (1/4 cup) Jarlsberg
  Lite cheese, grated

1 ripe plum tomato, sliced
2 ounces skinned turkey
  breast, fully cooked and
  sliced
nonstick cooking spray
1 cup watermelon chunks

Spread the mustard on each slice of bread. Put 2 tablespoons of cheese, the tomato and the turkey on one slice of bread. Sprinkle with the additional cheese and top with the remaining slice of bread. Grill the sandwich on a hot griddle or a nonstick skillet coated with nonstick spray. Cook until the bread is lightly browned and the cheese melts. Serve with the melon.

Makes 1 serving, giving 2 complex carbohydrates (the bread), 3 ounces protein (the turkey and the cheese) and 1 simple carbohydrate (the fruit).

Nutritional Profile per Serving
32 g carbohydrate; 29 g protein; 7 g fat; 20.5% calories from fat;
62 mg cholesterol; 551 mg sodium; 307 calories

Quick Mexican Chili

1 pound ground turkey
1 small onion, diced
1 small green pepper
1 can (15-1/2 ounces) tomato
 sauce
1 can (15-1/2 ounces) crushed
 tomatoes

1 can (15-1/2 ounces) kidney
 beans, rinsed
2 teaspoons chili powder
1 teaspoon garlic powder
1/2 teaspoon creole seasoning
1-1/2 cups brown rice,
 cooked

Crumble the ground turkey into a hard plastic colander. Microwave the turkey on high for 3 minutes; stir and break it apart. Add the onion and the green pepper. Microwave another 3 to 4 minutes until the turkey is browned. Spoon the meat and the vegetables into a saucepan and add the remaining ingredients. Cook the mixture over medium-high heat until it boils. Simmer uncovered for 10 more minutes, stirring to prevent it from burning.

Makes 6 servings (1-1/2 cups each). Serve over 1/4 cup cooked brown rice in a large soup bowl. Freeze the remaining servings in individual freezer bags for later use.

Each serving gives 1 complex carbohydrate (the rice), 3 ounces protein (the turkey and beans) and 1 simple carbohydrate (the veggies).

Nutritional Profile per Serving
32 g carbohydrate; 25 g protein; 1 g fat; 4% calories from fat;
47 mg cholesterol; 742 mg sodium; 237 calories

⋰ MAKE-IT-QUICK DINNERS ∿

 Sicilian Chicken and Pasta (*your protein, complex carbohydrate and simple carbohydrate*)
Marinated Cucumbers (*your healthy munchie*)

Sicilian Chicken and Pasta

4 boneless, skinless chicken breasts
1/2 teaspoon creole seasoning
1/2 teaspoon dried basil
1/2 teaspoon dried oregano
2 cans (15-1/2 ounces) Italian-style stewed tomatoes

2 tablespoons cornstarch
1/4 teaspoon Tabasco sauce
1 clove minced garlic
1/4 cup grated Parmesan cheese
1 small package of angel hair pasta (8 ounces)

Preheat the oven to 425 degrees. Sprinkle the chicken with the seasoning, and pat it with the herbs. Place the chicken in a baking dish, and cover it with foil. Bake for 15 minutes.

While the chicken is baking, pour the canned tomatoes into a medium saucepan and add the cornstarch, the Tabasco sauce and the garlic. Cook the mixture until it is thickened, about 5 minutes.

After 15 minutes, remove the chicken from the oven, pouring off any liquid from the pan. Pour the heated sauce over the chicken and sprinkle the grated cheese on top. Place the pan back in the oven and cook, uncovered, for 10 more minutes.

Cook the pasta according to the package directions. Drain and place it on a platter. Top the pasta with the chicken and the sauce.

Makes 4 servings, each giving 1 complex carbohydrate (the pasta), 3 ounces protein (the chicken and the cheese) and 1 simple carbohydrate (the tomatoes).

Nutritional Profile per Serving
27 g carbohydrate; 25 g protein; 9 g fat; 20% calories from fat;
50 mg cholesterol; 878 mg sodium; 396 calories

Marinated Cucumbers

4 cucumbers
1 small red onion, thinly
   sliced
1 teaspoon dried dill weed

1/2 cup no-oil Italian
   dressing
4 romaine or green leaf
   lettuce leaves

Wash and peel the cucumbers; slice in rounds. Add the onion slices and toss with the dill weed. Pour in the dressing and refrigerate at least 2 hours to blend the flavors. Serve on a lettuce leaf. Makes 8 servings of a healthy munchie.

Nutritional Profile per Serving
9 g carbohydrate; 1 g protein; 0 g fat; 0% calories from fat;
0 mg cholesterol; 280 mg sodium; 40 calories

2 Shrimp Creole (*your protein and complex carbohydrate*)
Steamed Broccoli (*your simple carbohydrate*)
Caesar Salad (*your healthy munchie and an added fat*)

Shrimp Creole

white wine Worcestershire sauce
1 pound fresh medium shrimp
nonstick cooking spray
2 teaspoons olive oil
2 cloves garlic, finely chopped
1 small red onion, finely chopped

1/2 teaspoon creole seasoning
2 cups tomato puree, canned
1/2 cup chicken stock, defatted
2 plum tomatoes, cut lengthwise into strips
2 cups brown rice, cooked
1 lemon wedge
sprinkle of fresh chopped herbs (such as basil or thyme)
2 cups broccoli, steamed

Marinate the shrimp in Worcestershire sauce for 1 hour. Spray nonstick skillet with nonstick cooking spray; heat with 2 teaspoons of olive oil. Add garlic and onions and sauté until they are softened and transparent. Season shrimp with creole seasoning and sauté quickly in the hot pan. Add tomato puree and chicken stock, heating through. Add tomato strips at the end of cooking.

Mound 1/2 cup rice in the center of each of four plates; spoon 1/4 of shrimp and sauce over each rice mound. Garnish with a lemon wedge and sprinkle with the chopped herbs. Serve with the steamed broccoli.

Makes 4 servings, each giving 1 complex carbohydrate (the rice), 3 ounces protein (the shrimp) and 2 simple carbohydrates (the tomato puree, the tomatoes and the broccoli).

Nutritional Profile per Serving
38 g carbohydrate; 23 g protein; 4 g fat; 14% calories from fat; 66 mg cholesterol; 357 mg sodium; 279 calories

Caesar Salad

4 cups romaine lettuce, washed and torn
1 clove minced garlic
1-1/2 tablespoons olive oil
1/2 teaspoon dry mustard
1 teaspoon Worcestershire sauce
1/8 teaspoon coarse black pepper

1/8 teaspoon salt (optional)
1 coddled egg*
juice of 1 lemon
1/4 cup Parmesan cheese, grated
croutons (from 2 slices whole wheat bread sprinkled with garlic powder and toasted till brown)

Rub the bottom and sides of a large salad bowl with the garlic; leave the garlic in the bowl. Add the oil, the mustard, the Worcestershire sauce and the spices; beat together with a fork or wire whisk. Add the chilled romaine lettuce; toss well. Crack the coddled egg over the salad; add the lemon juice and toss until the lettuce is well covered. Top with the Parmesan cheese and the croutons. Toss well and enjoy!

*Coddle an egg by immersing the egg in its shell in boiling water for 30 seconds. This makes it safe to eat.

Makes 6 servings, each giving 1 added fat.

Nutritional Profile per Serving
6 g carbohydrate; 4 g protein; 5 g fat; 51% calories from fat; 39 mg cholesterol; 152 mg sodium; 81 calories

③

Black Bean Soup Over Rice (*your protein and
complex carbohydrate*)
Spinach and Apple Salad (*your
simple carbohydrate*)

Black Bean Soup Over Rice

nonstick cooking spray
2 teaspoons olive oil
2 cloves garlic, finely
  chopped
1 small red onion, diced
2 cups chicken stock, defatted
4 cups cooked black beans (if
  canned, rinse and drain)

1 teaspoon creole seasoning
1 teaspoon ground cumin
2 cups brown rice, cooked
3 limes, halved
1 cilantro leaf (optional)

Spray a nonstick pan with nonstick cooking spray. Heat the
olive oil in the pan. Add the onion and the garlic; sauté until
translucent. Add the chicken stock, 2-1/2 cups of the cooked
black beans and the creole seasoning. Bring the mixture to a gentle
boil and cook until the amount is reduced by a third; puree in a
blender or food processor until smooth. (You may refrigerate this
now for serving later. Then reheat the bean puree; if necessary,
thin the puree with additional chicken stock to make it smooth.)

When serving, place 1/3 cup of the cooked brown rice in each
of 6 bowls. Top with 1/4 cup of the reserved whole black beans.
Add 1 cup heated bean puree. Squeeze 1/2 lime over each bowl.
Garnish with a cilantro leaf if desired.

Makes 6 servings, each giving 2 complex carbohydrates (the
rice), 2 ounces protein (the beans and the stock) and part of a
simple carbohydrate (the onion).

Nutritional Profile per Serving
47 g carbohydrate; 12 g protein; 3 g fat; 12% calories from fat;
0 mg cholesterol; 367 mg sodium; 261 calories

Spinach and Apple Salad

2 tablespoons canola oil
1-1/2 teaspoons basil
1 teaspoon onion powder
1/2 teaspoon salt (optional)
1/8 teaspoon pepper
3/4 cup apple juice

2 tablespoons apple cider
 vinegar
1/2 cup orange segments
4 cups spinach, torn in pieces
2 cups apple, thinly sliced

In a small bowl prepare the dressing by combining the oil, the basil, the onion powder, the salt and the pepper; set aside for 10 minutes to allow the flavors to blend. Stir in the apple juice and the vinegar. In a large bowl, combine the spinach, the apple and the oranges. Toss with 1/2 cup dressing; serve immediately. Refrigerate the remaining dressing for other salads or a marinade.

Makes 6 servings, each giving a simple carbohydrate.

Nutritional Profile per Serving
12 g carbohydrate; 1 g protein; 2 g fat; 26% calories from fat;
0 mg cholesterol; 30 mg sodium; 69 calories

Dijon-Crusted Salmon (*your protein*)
Baked Sweet Potato (*your complex carbohydrate*)
Green Beans With Mushrooms (*your simple carbohydrate and added fat*)

Dijon-Crusted Salmon

4 salmon fillets, 5 ounces
  each
white wine Worcestershire
  sauce to cover fish
nonstick cooking spray
1 teaspoon olive oil
1/2 teaspoon creole
  seasoning

4 tablespoons Dijon-style
  mustard
4 tablespoons toasted bread
  crumbs
2 tablespoons chopped fresh
  parsley

Marinate the fish in white wine Worcestershire sauce for at least 15 minutes to 1 hour. Preheat oven to 350 degrees. Spray a nonstick skillet with nonstick cooking spray and heat it with the olive oil. Sprinkle the marinated fish with creole seasoning and sear it quickly in the hot pan. Spread the top of each fillet with 1 tablespoon mustard; then sprinkle on 1 tablespoon bread crumbs and 1/2 tablespoon chopped parsley. Place the fillets in the hot oven and roast until they are browned and done, approximately 8 to 10 minutes.

Makes 4 servings, each giving 3 ounces protein.

Nutritional Profile per Serving
6 g carbohydrate; 25 g protein; 8.8 g fat; 39% calories from fat;
42 mg cholesterol; 434 mg sodium; 207 calories

Baked Sweet Potatoes

2 medium sweet potatoes   cinnamon (optional)

Preheat oven to 400 degrees. Wash and scrub 2 sweet potatoes. Place them on the oven rack, baking for 45 minutes or until fork tender. Or prick the scrubbed sweet potatoes with a fork, and microwave on high for 4 minutes. Turn the sweet potatoes over and microwave another 4 minutes. When serving, cut the potatoes in half and fluff with a fork; sprinkle with cinnamon, if desired.

Makes 4 servings, each giving 1 complex carbohydrate.

Nutritional Profile per Serving
14 g carbohydrate; 1 g protein; 0 g fat; 0% calories from fat;
0 mg cholesterol; 6 mg sodium; 60 calories

Green Beans With Mushrooms

2 teaspoons olive oil
1 clove garlic, minced
1/2 pound fresh
   mushrooms, washed
1/2 teaspoon dried rosemary
1/2 teaspoon dried basil

1 tablespoon dried parsley
1/2 teaspoon salt (optional)
1/4 teaspoon pepper
2 pounds green beans,
   steamed

Spray a nonstick pan with nonstick cooking spray. Sauté the garlic and mushrooms in olive oil for 5 minutes. Add the spices and simmer covered for another 3 to 4 minutes. Toss well with the beans.

Makes 6 servings, each giving 1 simple carbohydrate and an added fat.

Nutritional Profile per Serving
9 g carbohydrate; 2 g protein; 2 g fat; 17% calories from fat;
0 mg cholesterol; 4 mg sodium; 129 calories

Snapper With Tomato and Feta Cheese (*your protein*)
Corn on the Cob (*your complex carbohydrate*)
Cabbage Slaw (*your healthy munchie*)

Snapper With Tomato and Feta Cheese

2 ripe tomatoes, sliced
2 cloves garlic, finely minced
1 pound red snapper fillets
  (1/2" thick)

1 teaspoon dried basil
1 lemon, thinly sliced
1/2 teaspoon dried oregano
1/3 cup feta cheese, crumbled

Arrange the tomato slices on the bottom of a 9-inch glass pie dish. Sprinkle the garlic over the tomatoes and arrange the fish over the top. Sprinkle the basil over the fish. Place the lemon slices on top; sprinkle with the oregano and the crumbled feta cheese. If possible, let the fish sit for about 30 minutes.

Cover the fish with vented plastic wrap and microwave on high for 4-1/2 to 5 minutes. Let it stand for 5 minutes.

Makes 4 servings, each giving 4 ounces protein (the fish and the cheese) and half a simple carbohydrate (the tomatoes).

Nutritional Profile per Serving
7 g carbohydrate; 27 g protein; 6 g fat; 28% calories from fat; 60 mg cholesterol; 318 mg sodium; 190 calories

Cabbage Slaw

3 cups shredded cabbage
1 cup shredded red cabbage
1 cup shredded carrot
1/4 cup finely chopped onion
1/4 cup rice-wine vinegar

1/4 cup unsweetened
  pineapple juice
1 tablespoon Dijon-style
  mustard
1/8 teaspoon salt
1/8 teaspoon pepper

Combine the cabbages, the carrot and the onion in a medium bowl; toss gently. Combine the vinegar with the remaining ingredients and stir well. Add to the cabbage mixture and toss gently. Cover and chill at least 1 hour.

Makes 8 servings (1/2 cup each), each giving half a simple carbohydrate.

Nutritional Profile per Serving
5 g carbohydrate; 1 g protein; 2 g fat; 43% calories from fat;
0 mg cholesterol; 124 mg sodium; 42 calories

Turkey Burgers (*your protein and
complex carbohydrate*)
Raw Veggies With Yogurt Dip
(*your healthy munchie*)
Watermelon Quarters (*your simple carbohydrate*)

Turkey Burgers

3 pounds ground turkey breast	2 tablespoons minced garlic
8 ounces refrigerated hash browns or shredded raw potato	1/3 cup diced white onions
	4 ounces chicken stock, defatted
1/4 cup chopped parsley	2 egg whites or 1/4 cup egg substitute
1 tablespoon creole seasoning	whole wheat hamburger buns

Crumble the turkey into a bowl. Spray a nonstick pan with nonstick cooking spray; heat. Add the shredded hash browns and brown. Let the hash browns cool and then add them to the turkey with the remaining ingredients. Shape into 10 patties. Grill the patties and serve on whole wheat hamburger buns. The remaining patties may be frozen individually in freezer bags, before or after cooking. If the patties are frozen uncooked, thaw them in the refrigerator before grilling.

Each patty on a bun gives 2 complex carbohydrates (the potatoes and the buns) and 4 ounces protein (the turkey and the eggs).

Nutritional Profile per Serving
36 g carbohydrate; 30 g protein; 6.5 g fat; 19% calories from fat;
96 mg cholesterol; 244 mg sodium; 330 calories

Raw Veggies With Yogurt Dip

1 cup skim milk
1/2 cup nonfat plain yogurt
2 tablespoons dried minced
    onion
2 tablespoons lemon juice
1/2 teaspoon garlic powder

1/2 teaspoon salt (optional)
1/2 teaspoon dried oregano
1 teaspoon dried parsley
1/2 teaspoon onion powder
1/4 teaspoon black pepper
raw vegetables

Mix all the ingredients for the dip together and chill. Serve with raw vegetables.

Makes 12 1-ounce servings of 2 tablespoons each; this is a healthy munchie.

Nutritional Profile per Serving
1 g carbohydrate; 1 g protein; 0 g fat; 0% calories from fat;
0 mg cholesterol; 107 mg sodium; 12 calories

Zesty Chicken Quesadillas (*your protein and complex carbohydrate*)
Sliced Melon (*your simple carbohydrate*)

Zesty Chicken Quesadillas

4 10" whole wheat flour tortillas

4 skinless, boneless chicken breasts or 2 cans (6-1/2 ounces each) of white-meat chicken

1 yellow, red or green pepper

2 tomatoes, diced

4 ounces part-skim cheddar cheese, grated

2 ounces mixed greens: romaine, red leaf, Bibb

1 cup cooked black beans, (if canned, rinse)

1/4 cup picante sauce

cantaloupe, peeled and sliced

Cut the chicken breasts into lengthwise strips and poach or grill until tender. If using canned chicken, drain the 2 cans of white-meat chicken. Dice the peppers. Lay the tortilla in a large, heated nonstick skillet. Sprinkle 1/4 of the chicken breast strips, the diced peppers, the diced tomatoes and the cheese on one half of each tortilla. Fold over the other half of the tortilla and grill until it is browned and crispy and the cheese is melted.

Cut each quesadilla into 3 triangles and lay each piece on a plate next to the greens. Top the greens with the black beans. Serve with picante sauce for dipping. Lay cantaloupe slices to the side of the plate.

Makes 4 servings, each giving 2 complex carbohydrates (the tortilla), 4 ounces protein (the chicken, the cheese and the beans) and 1 simple carbohydrate (the veggies and the melon).

Nutritional Profile per Serving
40 g carbohydrate; 32 g protein; 10 g fat; 23% calories from fat;
66 mg cholesterol; 751 mg sodium; 385 calories

◡: For the Cook of the House :◡

Breaking the Tasting Chain

A cook often eats unconsciously. While cooking or cleaning, it's easy to pop in a taste of this, a bite of that, a little more of this and a spoonful of that. But all those "tastes" can add up to an entire meal's worth of calories! While cleaning the table, we fight our childhood warnings about wasting food. ("You need to clean your plate to help the starving children in Asia.")

Here are several tips to help you break the "tasting chain."

- If you feel you must taste the dish you are preparing so you can adjust the spices, keep a measuring teaspoon available for this purpose. This will limit the amount you test. Keep track of the exact measure of which spices you add to a recipe. Once you get a recipe just right, record exactly how much you used. Next time you will be able to trust the recipe without taste-tasting it.

- Cleaning up after a meal can cause as much harm as cooking it. Mom wasn't exactly giving you the facts when she said that cleaning your plate would save the lives of starving children. Your unhealthiness from overeating has never helped the hunger effort. If you want to aid those children, send money or support a charity. Do not overeat! Think of it this way: Wasting food is wasting food, whether in a body that doesn't need it or in a trash can. The difference: It doesn't hurt the trash can, but it does hurt your health.

- To make matters easier, serve up food at the stove, not family style, which leads to the clean-out-the-bowl habit and makes portion control difficult. Seal leftovers and put them away before you sit down to eat. Going for more requires more effort. *Leave a few bites on your plate* to put a dent in the clean-plate syndrome.

Time-Saving Tips

Few people these days have the time or inclination to spend every afternoon preparing the dinner meal. Actually, lack of time can be a major obstacle to a wellness strategy. If your philosophy is "If it takes longer to cook it than to eat it, forget it!" then these tips are for you.

- When you cook, do so in abundance, then freeze properly portioned leftovers in freezer bags, providing quick meals when you need them.

- Keep two empty shoeboxes in your freezer to store ready-made meals. Put main-dish portions in one box, complements to the meal (rice, pastas, vegetables) in the other box.

- Spend one hour each week preparing some of the basics that will make each night's meal a healthy delight with a minimum of effort. For example, cook a big pot of brown rice, which can be reheated as needed. Make a batch of tomato sauce for use with pasta or as a topping for meat or pita pizzas. Cook a pot of beans for beans and rice.

- For extra-quick stir-fry, use frozen bags of assorted vegetables. The vegetables are already precut and can be fully cooked in four minutes! Bags of frozen peas can also be used for a quick carbohydrate.

- For basic, quick salads, tear romaine lettuce and top with tomato, no-oil Italian dressing and a sprinkle of Parmesan.

- Keep raw veggies marinating in no-oil Italian dressing for a quick salad. Add a small can of tuna to make a main dish and cooked pasta to make a whole meal.

Use the following grocery list to guide you when you shop.

⌁ PAM SMITH'S ⌁
HEALTHY GROCERY LIST

GRAINS
Brown Rice: ❑ Instant
 ❑ Long-grain ❑ Short-grain
❑ Wild Rice
❑ Cornmeal
❑ Whole Wheat Bagels
❑ Whole Wheat Bread — 100%
(*first word of ingredients: "whole"*)
❑ Whole Wheat English Muffins
❑ Whole Wheat Hamburger Buns
Whole Wheat Pasta: ❑ Elbows
 ❑ Flat ❑ Lasagna ❑ Spaghetti
 ❑ Spirals
❑ Whole Wheat Pastry Flour
❑ Whole Wheat Pita Bread
❑ _____
❑ _____

CEREALS (*whole grain and less than 5 grams of added sugar*):
❑ Cheerios
❑ Grape-nuts
❑ Grits
❑ Muesli
❑ Nutri Grain Almond Raisin
Oats: ❑ Old-fashioned
 ❑ Quick-cooking
Puffed Cereals: ❑ Rice
 ❑ Wheat
❑ Raisin Squares
❑ Shredded Wheat
❑ Shredded Wheat 'N Bran
Unprocessed Bran: ❑ Oat
 ❑ Wheat

❑ Wheatena
❑ _____
❑ _____

CRACKERS
Crispbread: ❑ Kavli ❑ Wasa
❑ Crispy Cakes
❑ Harvest Crisps 5-Grain (*not all whole grain, but good for variety*)
❑ Rice Cakes
❑ Ry-Krisp
❑ _____

DAIRY
❑ Butter
Cheese (*low-fat — less than 5 grams of fat per ounce*):
Cheddar:
 ❑ Kraft Light Naturals
 ❑ Weight Watchers Natural
❑ Cottage Cheese 1%
❑ Farmer's
❑ Jarlsberg Lite
Cream Cheese:
 ❑ Philadelphia Light (*tub*)
 ❑ Philadelphia Fat free
Mozzarella: ❑ Nonfat
 ❑ Part-skim
 ❑ String Cheese
Nonrefrigerated:
 ❑ Laughing Cow Light
❑ Parmesan
Ricotta: ❑ Nonfat
 ❑ Part-skim
❑ Egg Substitute

- ❏ Egg Substitute
- ❏ Eggs
- ❏ Fleischmann's Squeeze Spread
- ❏ Milk (*skim or 1%*)
- ❏ Nonfat Plain Yogurt
- ❏ Stonyfield Farm Yogurt
- ❏ _____
- ❏ _____

CANNED GOODS
Chicken Broth: ❏ Swanson's
   Natural Goodness
Soups:
   ❏ Pritikin
   Progresso: ❏ Black Bean
      ❏ Lentil
Tomatoes: ❏ Paste ❏ Sauce
      ❏ Stewed ❏ Whole
- ❏ _____
- ❏ _____
- ❏ _____

FRUITS
- ❏ Apples ❏ Apricots ❏ Bananas
- ❏ Berries ❏ Citrus ❏ Cherries
- ❏ Dates (*unsweetened, pitted*)
- ❏ Grapes ❏ Kiwi
- ❏ Lemons ❏ Limes ❏ Melon
- ❏ Nectarines ❏ Peaches
- ❏ Pears ❏ Pineapple
- ❏ Plums ❏ Raisins
- ❏ _____
- ❏ _____
- ❏ _____

VEGETABLES
- ❏ Asparagus ❏ Broccoli
- ❏ Cabbage ❏ Carrots
- ❏ Cauliflower ❏ Celery ❏ Corn
- ❏ Cucumbers ❏ Green Beans
- ❏ Greens ❏ Kale
- ❏ Mushrooms ❏ Onions ❏ Peas
- ❏ Peppers ❏ Red Potatoes
- ❏ Romaine Lettuce ❏ Spinach
- ❏ Squash ❏ Sweet Potatoes
- ❏ Tomatoes ❏ White Potatoes
- ❏ Zucchini
- ❏ _____
- ❏ _____
- ❏ _____

BEANS AND MEATS
Beans and Peas: ❏ Black
   ❏ Chick-peas/Garbanzo Beans
   ❏ Kidney ❏ Lentils ❏ Navy
   ❏ Pinto ❏ Split Peas
- ❏ _____
Beef (*lean*): ❏ Deli-sliced
   ❏ Ground Round
   ❏ Round Steak
- ❏ _____
Fish and Seafood:
   ❏ Fresh ❏ Frozen
- ❏ _____
Lamb: ❏ Leg ❏ Loin Chops
Poultry:
   Chicken: ❏ Boneless Breasts
      ❏ Parts ❏ Whole Fryer
- ❏ _____
   Turkey: ❏ Breast ❏ Ground
      ❏ Sliced ❏ Whole
- ❏ _____
Veal: ❏ Chuck ❏ Leg Chops
   ❏ Loin Chops ❏ Round
   ❏ Rump ❏ Shoulder Chops
Water-packed Cans: ❏ Chicken
   ❏ Salmon ❏ Tuna
   ❏ Charlie's Lunch Kit
- ❏ _____
- ❏ _____

MISCELLANEOUS

All-Fruit Jam and Pourable
Syrup:
- ❑ Knudsen
- ❑ Polaner's
- ❑ Smucker's Simply Fruit
- ❑ Welch's Totally Fruit

Bean Dips
- ❑ Guiltless Gourmet

Boullion Cubes: ❑ Beef
- ❑ Chicken

Cooking Oils:
- ❑ Canola ❑ Olive
- ❑ Cornstarch

Fruit Juices (*unsweetened*):
- ❑ Apple ❑ Apple-Cranberry
- ❑ White Grape ❑ Orange

Garlic: ❑ Cloves ❑ Minced
- ❑ Honey

Mayonnaise: ❑ Light
- ❑ Miracle Whip Light
- ❑ Mustard
- ❑ Nonstick Cooking Spray

Nuts/Seeds (*dry-roasted,
unsalted*): ❑ Peanuts
- ❑ Sunflower Kernels

Pasta Sauce: ❑ Pritikin
- ❑ Ragu Chunky Gardenstyle
- ❑ Peanut Butter (*natural*)

Popcorn:
- ❑ Orville Redenbacher's
  Light Natural Microwave
- ❑ Plain Kernels

Salad Dressing:
- ❑ Bernstein's Low Calorie
- ❑ Good Seasons ❑ Kraft-Free
- ❑ Pritikin
- ❑ Soy Sauce (*low sodium*)

Spices & Herbs: ❑ Allspice
- ❑ Basil ❑ Black Pepper
- ❑ Cayenne Pepper
- ❑ Celery Seed ❑ Chili Powder
- ❑ Cinnamon ❑ Curry
- ❑ Dill Weed ❑ Garlic Powder
- ❑ Ginger ❑ Mustard
- ❑ Nutmeg ❑ Oregano
- ❑ Onion Powder ❑ Paprika
- ❑ Parsley ❑ Rosemary

Tortilla Chips/Baked Tostitos
- ❑ Guiltless Gourmet
- ❑ Vanilla Extract

Vinegars: ❑ Balsamic ❑ Cider
- ❑ Red Wine ❑ Tarragon
- ❑ White Wine Worcestershire
  Sauce

- ❑ _____
- ❑ _____
- ❑ _____

⌁ Tips for the Food Shopper ⌁

- Be sure to go shopping *after* you've eaten your healthy meal or snack. Do not go to the grocery store with your blood sugars low and your appetite out of control.

- Make a list of what you plan to buy — and stick to that plan. If it's not on the list, it doesn't belong in your cart. Let grocery shopping be a time to look for foods that *benefit* your body.

- Don't buy health-robbing foods "for the family." If you don't eat them on the way home, you will probably hide them in the back of the cupboard and eat them later. I can say from experience that these foods never seem to get past the hands of the buyer.

- Resist the temptation to feed others the very foods you are choosing to avoid. Feeding your loved ones energy-robbing, health-robbing foods is not an appropriate expression of love. You are only contributing to their unhealthiness.

Building Healthy Children

All parents want their kids to be good eaters — to eat their vegetables, grow up healthy and develop good eating habits while they are young.

You are your child's teacher. If you make poor food choices, you can expect your child to do the same. If your three-year-old sees his daddy pouring salt all over his food, then he, believing that Daddy is better than Superman, will learn to oversalt his food too. If Mom doesn't like fish and never serves it to her angel, her child will grow up thinking it's yucky. If big sister eats a PopTart everyday for breakfast, it won't be long before little sister will be doing the same.

Children who eat healthy foods when they're young are more likely to keep the habit as teens and adults. If you want to encourage wholesome snacking, don't munch on cookies or a bag of chips. If you don't eat breakfast, don't expect your child to either. If you have an aversion to a certain food, particularly a healthy one, keep it to yourself.

Remember that your attitudes about eating are a significant contribution to your little one's health. If you binge when you are stressed, bribe your kids with food or punish them by denying it, then you're putting an emotional charge on eating.

The long-term result is an improper relationship with food, one of the root causes of eating disorders. Instead, we can aspire to teach a healthy attitude about healthy food. Eating is enjoyable, satisfies hunger and meets the nourishment needs of our bodies, but it isn't meant to be the light of our lives.

Your children may not always do as you say, but you can be sure they will do as you do.

NINE

STRESS IS A STRETCH THAT WILL MAKE YOU SNAP OR MAKE YOU STRONG!

STRESS IS THE unavoidable price of modern life. Nearly nine out of ten Americans say they experience high levels of stress at least once or twice a week, and one in four complains of high levels every day. A common plea is, "If I can just get through this week (or this month or taxes or the end of school or this project), then things won't be so crazy."

The truth is, however, that something is always waiting around the bend for busy people. For me, although things don't get better, they don't necessarily get worse — they just get different!

Any dialogue about stress in the nineties also must include the guilt factor. Today's busy, overtired and overstressed men and women feel guilty about almost everything: not enough time spent with family and friends, unmade beds, messy garages and dirty dishes. We feel guilty about eating too much of the wrong things and too little of the right things, the shape of our bodies and getting too little exercise.

Statistics, as well as many personal testimonies, tell us that no one of any age is immune to stress.[1] We can surely use some new perspective in overcoming its effects.

Just as your body is designed to work for you nutritionally, it is also designed to survive the stresses of life — and can actually be strengthened by them.

The problem in treating stress is identifying and understanding it. Stress is one of those words that everyone knows the meaning of, but few can define. We are experts in what stresses us. And what's stressful to me may not be stressful to you. Our reactions to life events vary from person to person: What frazzles one may challenge and give vision to another.

Any change that requires you to adjust your way of doing things can cause stress, good or bad: retirement, the death of a loved one, a traffic jam, a missing set of keys, even a surprise visit from a friend. Research shows that the number of changing events in one's life doesn't affect health and well-being, but the response to those events does.[2]

Many of us refer to these upsetting life events as stress, but they are actually called *stressors*. Like a coffee cup, we all have a certain capacity for stress. Whether or not the coffee overflows when poured depends on the cup's size. Likewise, people who have a seemingly large capacity to deal with challenge may not "overflow" under stress.

But what happens when stress starts to spill over? As three-parted beings, we respond to stress spiritually, emotionally and physically. Our emotional and spiritual reactions depend on the emotional and spiritual atmosphere in which we live. If our spirits are thriving on faith, stress can push us to a new growth and vision. If our emotions are thriving on love and nurturing, stress can stretch us into new, healthy places.

The Body's Response

Unlike the varied emotional and spiritual responses, the physical response to stress is universal. It is set by an elaborate, innate programming. We were created to survive, and our physical bodies are finely tuned for adaptation in stressful encounters to assure that we do survive.

We are designed with stress sensors — similar to radar tracking equipment — in our brains. These are on a constant seek-and-find mission, looking for threats to our survival. When these sensors pick up stress signals, they recognize them as danger, just as if a grizzly bear had stepped across our path. Messages are sent throughout the body to prepare for fighting or fleeing the present danger — or to "play possum" and hope it goes away.

These messages cause the symptoms of stress. To allow for optimum defense, chemical reactions tell the body to go into a conservation mode. This state of conservation includes three predictable physical reactions that clearly affect the whole being.

1) *The body's metabolism slows,* storing excess energy for the fight or flight. This metabolic slowdown explains part of the quick weight gain that often accompanies stressful times. Whether or not we eat more when under stress, the stressed body does more damage with what comes in than the nonstressed body does. Research just released from Yale University shows that the extra weight gained in stressful times localizes in the abdominal region. When stress hits, adrenaline mobilizes fat all over the body, and another chemical, cortisol, takes what is not used and stashes it in the midsection.

The metabolic slowdown effect of stress also impacts gastrointestinal function through increased secretions of gastric acids and faulty motility. This reads constipation for some; gastritis, ulcerations, diarrhea, spastic colon or irritable bowel syndrome for others. Those prone to increased acidity often have difficulties "facing food" when stressed; they keep a low-grade "queaze" at all times and are prone to a vicious "the less I eat, the worse I feel, and thereby the less I eat" mode.

2) *The body's blood sugar dips,* stimulating an appetite for high-calorie foods that will provide needed energy. As the blood sugars fluctuate, energy and moods drop, but appetite soars.

Yes, there's a physical reason for getting tired and cranky in stressful times. And, yes, there's a physical reason for craving M & M's (compounded with the emotions asking for food to tranquil-ize the anxiety!). You may notice that the word *stressed,* spelled backward, is *desserts!*

3) *The body retains excess fluids,* keeping the systems lubricated and hydrated for the defense.

Blood pools in our muscles and extremities, and we store the fluids in the extra poundage in our abdominal area, making us feel bloated and sluggish.

Spurts of stress chemicals — adrenaline, cortisol and others — prime the body for action. The heart beats faster; blood pressure rises; the rate of breathing increases; muscles tense.

The fight-or-flight mode was intended to be a response to dan-ger. This surge of chemical reactions may have ensured our ances-tors' early survival when they faced their grizzly bears, but it can wear us down when it results from ever-present dangers that we try to grin and bear. We do not experience the resolution or release that comes with the fight or flight. And real threats are hard to identify in today's world. We are constantly adjusting to new situ-ations, new rules, new roles and new expectations — all triggering the stress response. It is interesting that the body's physical re-sponse to both positive and negative stress appears to be the same; the body can't discern the difference between weddings and funerals!

Some days we face intense, crisis-oriented stress. But some peo-ple live with a level of day-to-day stress that makes them feel chronically out of control to one degree or another. Chronic stress takes a particular toll on the body because, though it fluctuates, it never really goes away. Rather than fighting or protesting it in a healthy way, our bodies stay in the stress response with all its accompanying symptoms.

Bodies exposed to this kind of chronic, unresolved stress never have a chance to recover and break out of the fight-or-flight mode. Stuck in these chemical surges, we suffer headaches, backaches, temperomandibular joint syndrome (TMJ), sleep disturbances, anxiety, depression, arthritic pain, asthma, gastrointestinal upsets, skin disorders and weight and eating problems. (Not exactly the Abundant Life Club!) In fact, the American Institute of Stress reports that 75 percent to 90 percent of all doctor visits involve stress-related complaints.

Are You Stress-Sick?

Researchers have linked the emotions churned up by stress to specific illnesses. Intriguing research affirms age-old scriptural truths that chronic feelings of hopelessness or unforgiveness can affect the immune systems; it is like interior sabotage.[3]

Hormones released during stress-producing situations suppress the activity of immune-system cells, making us more susceptible to attack. Our stress response is the damaging factor.

Unprocessed emotions, particularly negative ones like bitterness and resentment, are especially threatening. For instance, doctors at the University of Ohio have shown that significant stress, such as loss of a loved one, can actually lower several of the major immune factors in your bloodstream. Other studies suggest that this type of stress can increase the risk of infection from a cold or virus or perhaps even more tragic diseases.[4]

Medical researchers in California, Florida and North Carolina have found that stress-induced irritability and unresolved anger may increase production of certain hormones that are responsible for reducing the body's ability to fight disease and can lead to higher blood pressure and more heart attacks.[5] Anxiety and fear often affect the digestive system, contributing to the development of ulcers, colitis and irritable bowel syndrome.

Most scientists would be awed at Solomon's wise words:

Anxiety in the heart of man causes depression (Proverbs 12:25, NKJV).

A relaxed attitude lengthens a man's life (Proverbs 14:30, TLB).

A cheerful heart is good medicine, but a crushed spirit dries up the bones (Proverbs 17:22).

It's a joy when science confirms the miracle of how our bodies are "fearfully and wonderfully made" (Psalm 139:14). Clearly, holding onto unresolved negative emotions works against us — activating a spiritual law that leaves us wide open for the fiery darts of sickness. We must learn to feel our feelings and release them. Denying or suppressing feelings lets them ferment and oppress us.

Lift Up the Stress Shield

As important as it is to identify how stress affects us, learning how to defuse life's stressors is even more critical. When your stress load weighs heavy, wise eating, exercise and rest will enable you to stand strong and will make all the difference in your ability to "ride the wave" of stress rather than drowning in its undertow.

Eating smart strengthens our barricades against attack; it feeds our stress-fighting army. The eat-right prescription: small meals of high-energy, whole grain carbohydrates and power-building, low-fat proteins complemented by brightly colored fruits and vegetables, at least every two and one-half to three hours.

Unfortunately, when stress comes in the front door, wise eating and exercise often go out the window. It is easy to get distracted from wellness principles. Good eating erodes to "catch as catch can," and "quick and easy" takes precedence over nutritious. Energy plummets, leaving little motivation for exercise. An exhaustive cycle begins: The greater our stress levels, the more unhealthy our eating habits are — which leads to fatigue. The more fatigued we become, the less we exercise. The less we exercise, the more fatigued — and stressed — we become.

Although we know that healthy eating and exercise make a difference, they seem like more time-robbers and add to the already long list of "shoulds."

If this sounds familiar, try transforming "shoulds" to "coulds." A strategy of good nutrition can provide a deflective shield against the symptoms of stress: As the body's metabolism slows, properly timed and balanced eating can gear it up. When the stress chemicals produce more gastric acids, smart eating can neutralize the acids and stabilize digestive function. As the blood sugars fluctuate more widely and wildly, the right foods at the right time can undergird them, keeping them even and high. When the body retains more fluids, adequate protein and fluid intake helps restore proper fluid balance.

Start by focusing on a step-by-step program. Let the "Seven Secrets for Keeping the Body Fit, Fueled and Free!" (page 36) become your action plan for effective and enjoyable living. Pay particular attention to these tips:

- *Start your day with breakfast.* Without it, you will fight an energy deficit all day.

- *Eat lean protein foods at every meal and snack.* Power proteins, such as fish and seafood, chicken, lean meats, skimmed milk, cheeses and yogurts and beans and peanuts strengthen your force shield against stress attacks. They also provide vitamin D, iron and zinc, which are vital for maintaining a healthy immune army. Look for lower-fat sources of protein and use little added fat. Studies are showing that as fat goes down, immune power goes up.[6]

- *Power snack.* It will keep your energy and concentration high by holding the metabolism and blood sugars at an even level.

- *Eat more colorful fruits and vegetables.* These are valuable sources of potassium and the water-soluble vitamins your body needs when fighting stress. Remember to shop for color. It means more nutritional power.
  Brightly colored fruits and vegetables, such as car-

rots, sweet potatoes, tomatoes, broccoli, spinach, romaine lettuce and strawberries, are loaded with beta-carotene and vitamin A, folic acid and other B vitamins, along with vitamin C. These nutrients help to stimulate the fighter-forces of our immune systems. Five servings a day will help to keep the doctor away!

- *Go for the grain.* Not only do these "staff of life" foods contain energy-giving carbohydrates, but they also supply vitamin B6, selenium and magnesium, all nutrients that are critical for activating the internal stress-fighting troops. They also contain fibers not found in many other foods. Look for breads, cereals and pastas made from whole grain flours.

- *Drink plenty of water.* It helps your body release the build-up of waste and fluid retained when the body faces stress.

Keep Your Sword Sharp

Properly timed and balanced eating can keep your energy level high and your body actively metabolizing the nutrients you eat. In addition, it energizes you for exercise and allows for more restful sleep, both of which serve as swords cutting away at stress. We need more than a deflective shield to offset the negative symptoms of stress; we need a sword and a shield!

The next two chapters cover the remaining body secrets for exercise and rest. Everyone knows these are a vital part of healthful living. But there's more to the story: They help to right the wrong of overstressed bodies.

Exercise is an offensive weapon in the war against stress. It's a *stress-buster!* As I have said, when sensing danger, the brain secretes chemicals that tell the body to fight or flee, setting into motion the symptoms of stress. But aerobic exercise, simulating the physical exertion inherent in the fight or flight, prompts the release of stress-busting chemicals called endorphins. Working somewhat like morphine, endorphins tell the body that it is no longer in danger. (You defeated or outran the grizzly!) You took control of the stressful situation; it no longer controls you.

Every time you walk, your body thinks you are fleeing your present danger; every tennis ball you hit tells your body that you've had your fight; ballroom dancing tells your body that you're waltzing away from the threat.

Nothing else can replace exercise; it is *the* key to responding positively to stress. This is why exercise is considered God's best tranquilizer. Exercising just thirty minutes a day is one of the best methods for releasing tension. It can also be your quiet time in the midst of a busy day, a time when you can divert and reflect on your true source of strength.

Ironically, when life is most stressful, when we have the least amount of time to exercise, rest and eat well, we need it most. But taking charge of our bodies is one thing we can control — we've been called to control — even in the midst of situations that feel very out of control.

Lighten Up

It is critical to realize that *there's no reason why stress should get the better of us.* Overcoming stress is seeing that, although we don't always get to choose our circumstances, we do have a choice in how we respond to them — as victims or victors.

We have to learn to lighten up. We get stressed and sick when we try to do too much or when we take ourselves too seriously. Stress is a sure sign we've taken our eyes off God and put our eyes onto our own strivings. Lining up our priorities — putting our time into the important, not just the urgent — releases incredible pressure.

Laugh, Brother, Laugh!

Incredibly, only one activity other than exercise produces the stress-busting endorphins: laughter!

Zig Ziglar calls laughter "internal jogging," and that's pretty close to the effect it has on the body. It is a mini-workout! Can you believe it? One hundred laughs a day provide a cardiovascular workout equivalent to ten minutes of rowing or biking, and laughter simulates a stress-release in the same way.

When you laugh you are telling your body that the stressful circumstance is no big deal! It can't be that bad if you can still laugh.

More words from Solomon: "A heart at peace gives life to the body" (Proverbs 14:30). Laughter even helps us fight infection by releasing hormones that can cut the immune-dampening effects of stress. Now that's something to laugh about!

The bottom line is that if we look after ourselves, our bodies will look after us. Taking care of ourselves is a small investment with tremendous returns. It does more than add years to our lives; it adds life to our years!

So the next time the enemy of life attempts a strike against you, lift up your shield, pick up your sharpened sword — and laugh in his face!

EXERCISE IS VITAL TO WELL-BEING

PROPER NUTRITION WITHOUT exercise is like a car without tires — the body may look good, but it won't go anywhere! Most of us know that exercise helps to right the wrongs of overstressed bodies. It gears up slowed metabolisms, improves muscle tone, helps to reduce blood pressure and puts the brakes on simple depression and stress. Exercise is *the* offensive tool to cut off the body's stress response.[1]

In addition to cutting the effects of stress on the body, moderate regular exercise keeps us well by strengthening the immune system over the long term. One study found that those who walked forty-five minutes a day, five days a week, had as much as a 57 percent increase in one kind of immune-cell activity and were half as likely to be sick with colds or flus as those who were not exercising. Because of what we know about exercise, many of us begin exercise programs. Some begin them every January 1; others, every Monday morning. Unfortunately, the knowledge that exercise is good for us doesn't seem to be enough to make us stick with it. As many as 80 percent of those who start an exercise routine drop out soon after starting. And only 40 percent of Americans exercise regularly, with only 20 percent reaping aerobic benefits. Clearly, we need some help in staying committed to a lifestyle of fitness.

Exercise for Undisciplined "Soles"

You can't store fitness; it's a daily choice. Your reward will be a strengthening of your armor: building up protective barriers against heart disease, diabetes, bone loss, arthritis, even cancer. In addition, regular exercise activates your metabolism. It allows the body to burst out of the cocoon, gearing up your calorie- and fat-burning potential by fanning the metabolic fire.

In addition to burning calories, exercise gives you an "after burn." It boosts your metabolism so you use up more calories for hours after you finish your workout.

And exercise is not only good for the body; it's great for the soul. It increases self-esteem, improves general appearance and gives you a wonderful sense of well-being.

Despite the benefits of exercise, it is nonetheless difficult to find a program you can stick to and enjoy. Consequently, many people have a history of start-and-stop exercising. Others consistently drive themselves to work out but derive little pleasure from it. Still others simply avoid exercise altogether. If you fall into one of these categories, odds are that you haven't found the exercise pattern that's right for you — or the energy to jump on the fitness bandwagon. To "just do it," you'll need to select an exercise that matches your lifestyle, your fitness needs and your personality.

◡ What Does Exercise Do for You? ◡

- Exercise increases metabolism and decreases appetite.

- Aerobic exercise increases your protection against heart disease by improving your heart's condition (making it more efficient) and increasing your HDL (high-density lipoproteins) cholesterol, the heart-protective form of cholesterol. Any exercise that raises your pulse to a training rate or, more simply, gets you breathing hard is an aerobic exercise. The benefits occur from achieving that increased pulse rate and maintaining it for at least twenty straight minutes three times a week. It is recommended that you gradually increase your exercise time up to an hour every other day.

- Exercise breaks the plateaus or set points of weight loss. It is an external way of boosting the metabolism naturally lowered in the body's attempt to maintain a certain weight.

- Exercise is nature's best tranquilizer. Exercising thirty minutes a day is one of the best ways of releasing tension. Exercise is *the* healthy outlet for stress — certainly a more acceptable alternative to eating, drinking or smoking!

- Recent studies have shown that exercise seems to be a vital factor in promoting excellent bone growth and lifelong maintenance. A well-planned exercise routine may stimulate the development of strong bone mass and later slow down any bone loss resulting from osteoporosis. Exercise increases the circulation and flow of nutrients to the bone, encouraging new bone growth and repair. Without routine exercise, bones may shrink, weaken and become porous.

The best exercises to build strong bones are the weight-bearing type, such as brisk walking, jumping rope and bicycling. As bones are stressed from these activities, they become stronger and denser. Swimming, although an excellent aerobic exercise, is not as effective in strengthening bones. To prevent and reduce the effects of osteoporosis, it is recommended that a person exercise at least every other day for twenty-five to thirty minutes.

If you are ready to join the ranks of those who successfully develop — and enjoy the benefits of — a regular exercise routine, take note: You don't have to take up the latest exercise craze to become fit.

Instead you can forge your own path, at your own pace and in your own direction. The frequency, intensity and duration of your workouts will influence the extent of the health benefits you reap. The type and time of exercise you choose will determine whether you stick with it.

↶ Exercise Guide to Be F.I.T.T. ↷

Frequency: four to six days a week.

Intensity: at a level where you feel slightly out of breath, without gasping. Exercise should not hurt. If something hurts, stop and rest. If the pain persists, check with your doctor. "No pain, no gain" is an exercise lie.

Exercising less than these guidelines recommend will produce some benefit but not enough. Exercising more may be useful for athletic training, but it can lead to injury.

How often and how hard to exercise are frequent questions. The answer always depends upon the individual's goals. A person actively seeking fitness needs to exercise four to six times per week. A person working to maintain good fitness should exercise three or four times each week. And someone under intensive stress may need some form of exercise every day, since it is the physical way to process that stress effectively. When your life is most stressful — when you have the least amount of time to exercise — you will gain the most from it.

The key to exercise is not to let it become stressful. Too much, too hard, has been shown to impair immunities and lead to vulnerability to injuries.

It takes a lot of exercise to make this happen — two to three hours of hammering the body — much more than most of us would do. Moderation in all things, even exercise, is the age-old word of wisdom.

Time: thirty to sixty minutes, at a time of day you feel good and your schedule allows routine to be built.

Choose the time of day that suits your schedule. Is it early morning? This is a great choice for beating the heat, and you won't be interrupted by schedule surprises as easily as you might be later in the day. (Those who begin exercising in the morning are more likely to be at it a year later.)

Suggestion: Set your alarm to get up, get dressed for a walk, bike ride or run, and just do it! As you're walking out the door, have energy-boosting juice first (four to six ounces of apple, white grape or unsweetened cranberry juice will do), then eat breakfast as soon as you come in.

If you choose midday as your exercise time, find an indoor activity to protect you from the heat. Exercising in over 90-degree weather is not a wise idea for anyone. And anytime you are active in the heat, be sure you are giving your body lots of water to replace the fluids you are losing to perspiration. You need at least six ounces of water for every twenty minutes of exercise.

Is early evening your best time? Although you have to guard this time (it's easy to skip your workout after hectic workdays), it's a tremendous time to take advantage of the appetite-suppressing and stress-releasing power of exercise. By diverting from your day's activities, you can downshift from stress to relaxation. I use this as a time to review my day — the good, the bad and the ugly — and get a pulse on how I feel about the things that occurred.

If you exercise later in the evening, your best bet is half an hour after dinner. Exercise substantially increases the number of calories burned to digest your food and improves how your body utilizes the nutrients from the meal. And you can enjoy the twilight cool and maybe even catch a gorgeous sunset! The majesty of a sunset always speaks to my struggles, which seem so small when I get a glimpse of God's work.

Type: Whatever type of aerobic exercise you enjoy (or could enjoy) and can do regularly.

Basically, three types of exercise are needed to provide the best workout and to work all the muscles of your body: warm-up, conditioning and aerobic exercise. Use warm-up exercises such as light side-to-side movements to limber up muscles and to prevent injuries from the other types of exercise.

Conditioning or strengthening exercises are those that tone the muscles through repetitive movements. Either handheld weights or a weight machine can be used to shape and define the muscles. Building muscle mass is not just a good idea for body builders; it's a terrific way to boost ailing metabolisms. In 1993 researchers at King's College, University of London, found that people with more muscle burned more calories constantly, even while they were sleeping. They found that those who weight-trained moderately for about an hour a day burned about 8 percent more calories than sedentary people. Really athletic types who trained harder and longer burned 14 percent more calories around the clock.

Experts agree that the most crucial exercises are the aerobic ones — those that work the heart and the circulatory systems. The major aerobic activities are walking, running, jumping rope, swimming and aerobic dancing. These exercises all use major muscle groups, burn fat and help keep the body working efficiently. You can choose one or a combination of all, but you're most apt to stick with the ones you find the most fun.

For those of us who don't think any exercise is fun; who cringe at the thought of jogging; who can't easily get to a pool for swimming; who don't have the time, place or desire for aerobic dancing, there is an alternative.

Brisk walking. It works the very best for me.

A Fitness Alternative

Fitness walking can be even more beneficial than more vigorous exercising, if it's done correctly. Walking just may be the exercise program you've been looking for! It's structured, simple, easy, quick and cheap — and is guaranteed to make you feel better and look better in just a couple of weeks.

Studies over the past few years have shown walking to be more effective in weight loss than heart-thumping runs. And a recent study at the Cooper Aerobics Center found that three-mile-a-day walkers ambling along at a twenty-minute-a-mile pace burned more fat than those going at a quicker twelve-minute-a-mile pace. The slower walk draws from the fat stores in the body rather than the muscle stores of energy.

I can walk in my neighborhood or anywhere business takes me. I can walk at the time of day that best fits my schedule and when the weather best suits a walk.

I have periodically tried other forms of exercise, such as aerobics classes and racquetball and health clubs, and I ran for many years, but walking is the form that now fits me best.

Find those minutes in the morning (before breakfast) or after work (ideally, before dinner or thirty minutes afterward) to go for a brisk walk around your neighborhood. If you are traveling or don't feel comfortable walking in your own neighborhood, stop off on the way home in an area where you feel safe. Just remember to pack your walking shoes! Look for a shoe that offers stability, good arch support and durability, with a half-inch maximum heel height. The heel should be rolled and tapered. Combine good shoes with good-quality athletic socks that fit smoothly and evenly on your feet.

Newcomers to fitness walking should measure off a mile and

walk it briskly. Walk fast enough to work up a light sweat (swing your arms and take long, but comfortable strides), but not so fast that you become breathless. This is your ideal aerobic pace. You should always be able to talk to a companion (or hum to yourself) during exercise. If you can't do this, slow your pace.

How long did it take you to walk that mile? Gradually increase your pace till you are walking it in fifteen minutes. Now add a second mile and work up to a pace of two miles in thirty minutes. Then add a third mile and work till you can walk the three miles in forty to forty-five minutes.

Before and after each walk, gently stretch to keep muscle soreness and tightness to a minimum. Stretch your shin muscles, calf muscles and tendons, hamstrings and front thighs with a slow, steady pull until you feel the muscles slightly ache. Hold each stretch for fifteen seconds. Do these stretches even on days you don't exercise to keep your muscles from tightening.

By warming up your muscles — stretching them, then beginning your exercise at a slow pace — you help prevent injuries. Cooling down — slowing down the exercise pace, then finally stretching the muscles — helps stop them from tightening up and cramping.

Plan on getting some walking in every day or at least four days a week. Within a few weeks your exercise program will be a habit, and you'll feel uncomfortable if you have to miss a day. And you'll clearly see and feel the benefits of more energy, better moods, more resiliency against stress and more restful sleep each night.

Know Yourself

The exercises you'll find most enjoyable will probably be those you feel you can best handle. If you have difficulty with eye-hand coordination, you may be frustrated by a sport like tennis but would do well with walking or swimming. If you are not naturally flexible, you may be happier with bicycling than ballet.

Consider the shape you are in. If you are overweight, any activity that involves pounding on your feet, such as running or aerobic dance, may stress your joints by placing too much weight on them.

Try riding a stationary bike or swimming instead.

If you're over thirty-five, most exercise experts encourage you to see a health professional for an all-points check before beginning an exercise program.

Try a Little Kindness

Think of exercise as an act of kindness to your body, not a punishment. Start slowly and avoid overtaxing yourself. The biggest exercise mistake people make is doing too much, too soon. Set realistic goals. Remember that exercise is a vital tool for fighting chronic stress and keeping your body fit and working for you. Let it be something you choose to do for life.

Get on those walking shoes and put your best foot forward!

ELEVEN

REST IS THE KEY TO RECHARGING

TO ENJOY LIFE spiritually, emotionally, relationally and physically, we must rest — in order to be recharged and renewed. If we don't take the time to rest, it's only natural for us to become depleted, sick and tired.

You may protest, "Recharge and rest — ha! You don't know my life; you don't understand the demands. I couldn't possibly squeeze out another moment!"

And you're right — I don't know your particular situation. But

I do know what happens when we are overcome with responsibilities and end up burned out, sometimes sick and sometimes bitter.

We see a role model for rest in Jesus; even He required quiet time to maintain His peace: "The news about him spread all the more, so that crowds of people came to hear him and be healed of their sicknesses. But Jesus often withdrew to lonely places and prayed" (Luke 5:15-16).

Rest for the Weary

How many of us fall into bed at night, "dead to the world" (or is it dead *from* the world?), seeking a few hours of relief from the hectic days of our lives? We are physically exhausted, emotionally weary and spiritually empty. Too many days of doing whatever it takes have taken their toll. Too many hours of getting through have gotten us. Bedtime comes, but refreshing sleep may not.

For some it's as difficult to turn off the day as it is to turn off the TV. There is simply too much to do and not enough time to do it, and robbing from sleep time seems to be an easy way to make up the difference.

Chances are you're in the same boat. Experts report a near epidemic these days of people who short themselves on sleep. Ask ten people how disciplined they are with a sleep schedule, and you'll be likely to hear variations on a single theme: "I go to bed when I finish doing what I have to do." You may even pick up on an attitude: Many are downright proud of undersleeping. Sleep loss is a macho power thing for many; getting by on four hours has a superhuman sound.

This isn't the problem for everyone; for many of us going to bed is a welcome respite and can even serve as an escape. The problem arises once we get there — and we don't rest.

The late hours designated for sleep can become a copy of our days; we fight through them. Tossing, turning, trying to count sheep, but counting our debts, tasks and tears instead.

Research still shows that we need seven to eight hours of deep, restful sleep a night.[1] Proper rest is a critical spoke in the wheel of wellness. Without it every aspect of bright, abundant living is dimmed. We are not at our effective and productive best. We don't have the energy to exercise. We don't look at life from a bright perspective. We don't even think as rationally or creatively as we should.

We may be living life in the nineties, but we still have the same bodies that need to live by the same principles God created long ago. In all of creation He models for us His principle — the need for rest. God created the soil of the earth to need a rest from time to time, allowing it to become more productive. Bears hibernate. The most beautiful plants have a period of dormancy. We can learn from these truths, and we can learn from Him: "So on the seventh day he rested from all his work" (Genesis 2:2).

We were created in His image, with a need to take time out to rest, to recreate, to reflect and to be regenerated.

Recognize the Need

Robbing ourselves of sleep, or being robbed of restful sleep, robs us of half our mental powers to carry us through the next day.[2] We then run on just a few cylinders. The symptoms can stay hidden though, because we're experts on coping. After awhile, sleepiness can even start to feel normal, and we forget what waking up feeling good is like.

The danger signs are subtle and easy to deny. We become grouchy; we're forgetful; our minds fog when forced to make quick decisions; we lose our sense of humor; and our creativity seems to lock up. Tests show that spontaneity, flexibility and originality in the thought process (all considered creative abilities) can be seriously undermined by as little as one sleepless night.[3]

Rest More and Sleep More

Making rest a lifestyle is choosing to give our cares to God in our waking hours as well as in our sleeping. We enter rest when we let go of all we don't want, won't use and don't need. We feel uplifted and drawn to the new because we aren't struggling to carry the old.

147

Once this becomes revelation, restful sleeping becomes part of an empowered lifestyle. The productivity it gives back to our days is well worth the hours invested.

In addition to the right quantity of sleep, we need good quality of sleep. Restful sleep is disturbance-free. Although it's normal to awaken briefly two to ten times per night — to shift position, for example — you won't remember these interruptions. But they can cut short the deepest, most refreshing stages of sleep and leave you groggy and grouchy the next day. Studies at the Henry Ford Sleep Disorders and Research Center in Detroit have found that being briefly disturbed every ten minutes throughout the night has the same effect as a three- to four-hour sleep loss.[4]

Here are some sleep tips to keep your body keyed for restful sleep:

Remember the fitness connection. Exercise helps you process the stresses of your day, allowing sweeter sleep. It is God's natural tranquilizer! No need to run marathons to get the benefits of exercise; just a walk, a bike ride or a swim can work wonders for your body — and your sleep.

Be clock-driven. Block in sleep as a priority part of your schedule. By doing this you are deciding in advance that sleep is important. When it comes to catching up on lost sleep, timing is everything.

The body's time clock is reset by getting up at the same time each day. For this reason, research shows that going to bed earlier in the evening offers an advantage over sleeping late the next morning; getting to sleep an hour earlier can provide the extra rest without upsetting the body's rhythm.[5] Stick with it; people who are just starting to make up lost sleep can take six weeks to recover fully.

Choose nighttime snacks wisely. Overeating or eating fat- or sugar-laden snacks after dinner can result in such an overload to the body that it will resist either getting to sleep or staying asleep.

The classic pattern is waking up from 2:30 A.M. to 3:00 A.M. with eyes open and heart racing, unable to get restfully back to sleep. Fluctuating blood sugars can bring you to such a light state of sleep that you are easily awakened. You may think it's the call of the bathroom — and this may be the case — but it may also be that bowl of ice cream or the chips or the cookies you ate just before going to bed!

A great bedtime snack is a small bowl of whole grain cereal with low-fat milk or yogurt. It keeps the body chemistries undergirded through the night, allowing you to awaken rested and refreshed.

If you do awaken too early — and your mind is stormed with cares and deadlines — the adrenaline pump turns on, dropping your blood sugars and keeping you awake. Bringing your blood sugars up with a small glass of juice will help to stabilize your chemistry and help get you back to a restful sleep.

If you drink caffeine-containing beverages (coffee, tea or cola-type sodas), recognize that the stimulant activity is still at work five to seven hours after you've ingested it. It may prevent your body from falling into deep sleep and can awaken you prematurely.

Minimize noise. Thick padding on floors and heavy drapes on windows help, as does a fan or air conditioner to make a steady background sound.

Rest more during the day. Often we don't rest well at night because we haven't taken enough time out during the day. We fall into bed exhausted, yet with so much adrenaline pumping through the body that we just can't relax and get to sleep. Letting renewal and recharge become a daily part of your life is a big step toward peaceful, restful sleep.

Time for Time-outs

How about time out for recharge and renewal? It is possible to find time for time-outs, even in the middle of busy lives and schedules. And you don't have to go away to do it. Here's how:

Schedule it. An obvious but often overlooked fact is that you have to make time for time out. In your hectic schedule of living, weekly carve out one hour (or longer!) for yourself — an hour in which you'll have nothing to do. Plan ahead for when the hour will be, but don't plan what you'll do; otherwise it will become one more thing on your to-do list. Permit yourself to lay aside the weight of responsibility for that period of time.

Start your day with it. Many of us have learned the power of starting the morning in a quiet time of reflection and connection with God. This is a daily part of my life, because I know that nothing is more important for me to do, and it's the only way I can start my day operating from strength. It is a time in the midst of my busy-ness to divert and reflect on who my source of strength really is. I often speak of it as being the warm-up for the exercise of my day; a time to stretch spiritually and get my heart circulating.

End your day with it. I'm now attempting to end my day with a time-out, a practice that is new to me — and difficult. I have to tell myself there is nothing else I should be doing. In this time-out I enjoy some of my favorite things, such as reading travel magazines, listening to favorite music or journaling. These activities don't seem productive in the scheme of life, yet I know they are vital in the scheme of my recharging.

It doesn't come naturally for me to do this; I'm a doer by nature. The first one up in our household, I go nonstop till the sun goes down and beyond. Even my breaks have a purpose: planning, researching, praying through my prayer list, meeting with my small group. I have laughed for many years about being a "human doing" rather than a human being. But only in recent years have I realized it's not something to laugh at.

Define your sabbath rest. Try using one day as a true time-out — a day of sabbath rest. Whether it's Sunday or another day, you need a weekly withdrawal. A day of rest for me means a day of activities that personally replenish me. It may mean time for reading novels, taking leisurely walks, napping, being with friends who recharge me, window shopping or just sitting and dreaming.

Something happens to me when I do this. I return to what I was created to be: a human being. I can review how I'm normally spending my time and if it's in line with the purposes to which I've been called. Otherwise, I stay too busy for issues of the heart.

Does this sound as if it's more the ideal than reality? It needn't be. It may seem impossible to carve out these personal moments of renewal. But with determination and a little creativity, you can put aside the time for joy and peace to be planted in your heart. "Freely you have received, freely give" (Matthew 10:8). It is a gift to yourself that becomes a gift to others — a gift that keeps on giving.

Abandon annually. Whether for a day, a weekend or a week, look for (and grab!) an opportunity to get away from the normal distractions of life. One of the most powerful gifts of wellness we can give ourselves is an annual abandon — leaving all the demands of daily life for a time for refreshment and renewed vision. Resist the temptation to schedule every moment with activities and people. Leave some time to make significant spiritual connections. Without the interruptions and the cares of this world this can be a quality time that recharges and revitalizes your soul. Recreation should be "re-creation," holding the promise of stretching your renewal right through the rest of the year!

TWELVE

WELLNESS
IS AN
INSIDE-OUT JOB

Y OU ARE WHAT you eat. This cliché is an oft-neglected but sobering thought for us — that what we are feeding our bodies affects what we are. The fuel we put in determines whether we thrive or just survive.

This realization is even more sobering when applied to our emotional and spiritual health. Are our responses to life's joys and heartaches a reflection of what's inside us?

As I mentioned in the introduction, I have found through my

years of counseling that eating well is not enough to make us well. More than caring for and feeding our physical beings, living well means caring for and feeding our souls — with the right kind of soul food. This means making peace with food, with our bodies, with our feelings and with God.

Soul Food

God has patterned an intricate design for our physical growth. No one is born an adult. We come into the world as tiny infants programmed for growth through nourishment. To grow and thrive, the human body requires certain nutrients; without them it becomes malnourished.

A similar design exists for our emotional growth.

At birth we are emotionally immature. We grow emotionally in much the same way we grow physically. If we are deprived of our emotional nutrients, our emotional growth is arrested, and we fail to thrive.

Even though our bodies may grow to physical maturity, our emotions can remain stunted. As adults we may appear to be coping with day-to-day life, but the child inside may be suffering from an overwhelming sense of shame, guilt, distrust or lack of confidence. When hit with adult stresses, hurts and challenges, our responses are often those of the emotionally disabled.

Picture it this way: As children our souls are planted with emotional seeds that grow as we grow. In a healthy family these seeds are unconditional love, respect and acceptance, and they later develop into beautiful blossoms of self-esteem and personal worth. We value who we are and learn to be confident, independent adults.

But not all families plant such healthy seeds of love into the souls of their children. Instead, some plant seeds of abandonment, wounding and shame. As children from these families grow into adulthood, these unhealthy emotional seeds grow into invisible weeds of guilt and fear, poor self-image, a false sense of obligation to others and lack of trust in God.

You cannot control what was planted in you as a child. You are not to blame for the wrong choices of other people, for the emotional food that was fed to you or for the lack of healthy soil in which you grew. These unhealthy seeds have certainly affected your life, but they have not ruined it. To thrive, not just survive, you must identify and root out these emotional weeds of your soul.

If you struggle with emotions you don't understand or can't release, you may need a healthy dose of "weed and feed." The roots of these destructive weeds are not killed easily. The enemy of life has fertilized them with lies, telling you change is hopeless.

But change *is* possible. You need to nourish your soul with Spirit-inspired "food" — the truth of who you are and why you were created. Knowing the truth about who you are is critical to your emotional well-being. It determines how you live, what you accomplish and how you treat — and are treated by — others.

The truth is that you are not a mistake. You were created by the God of the universe. You are an individual, highly unique and important, formed in the womb perfectly and specifically in His image (see Psalm 139:13-14; Genesis 1:26-27).

If you don't feel valuable, taking care of your body seems unimportant. It will be easy, then, to get caught in destructive patterns of eating. If you think you are junk, you will eat junk food.

Once you see yourself as valuable, you will take care of yourself. You are worth it! And you deserve to be happy and healthy.

Healing Feelings

As you start taking care of yourself and nourishing your physical body, many emotions that food, overeating, starving or dieting have helped you *submerge* will likely *emerge*. New feelings may bubble to the surface. These feelings need to be processed in new, healthy ways to prevent them from becoming logjams to your wellness. Processing your feelings requires that you understand how you are made — as an emotional being who feels feelings.

Many of us have grown up in families that discouraged both recognizing and expressing feelings, particularly negative ones such as anger, guilt or frustration. In these families children quickly learn which feelings get positive or negative reactions from parents. Life becomes a list of emotional shoulds and should nots: "You shouldn't feel that way." "You should be happy with what you have." "You shouldn't think of yourself all the time." This leaves us with the impression that what we feel is bad, wrong or unacceptable. But we are humans, created to feel. Birds fly; fish swim; humans feel!

Even if we judge our feelings as bad and deny or "stuff" them — often with food — they don't go away. When feelings are repressed, they linger and grow stronger, becoming a driving force in our lives.

To face or embrace feelings means to feel those emotions we have denied or suppressed — perhaps for a lifetime. But not to feel or express our feelings just causes them to come out in other ways, even making us sick. They may exit through headaches, joint and muscle pain, or an inability to sleep.

Instead of crying, we might get headaches. Instead of saying we don't want to be with someone, we might get stomach cramps. Instead of saying no to another project, we might push ourselves to exhaustion and develop high blood pressure — or we overeat. Our bodies react whether we like it or not. The unreleased energy robs us of our well-being by causing increased tension, anxiety or depression. Depression is considered emotion that has been frozen, which brings a rush of oppression.

If we shut down our emotions altogether, the brain produces chemicals that appear to suppress the activity of immune-system cells, making us more susceptible to infections and disease (see "Are You Stress-Sick?" on pages 130 and 131). Unprocessed feelings like fear, bitterness and resentment keep us bound to a spiritual hopelessness — a particularly threatening place to live. This kind of emotional condition produces a "possum" stress-reaction — we give up and play dead. Numbing our emotions causes the brain to secrete a chemical called cortisol. Cortisol is a hormone that plays havoc with our immune system, decreasing the function of our T-cells, the warriors that fight off disease.

FOOD FOR LIFE

Let Off Some Steam

Emotions produce energy. Remember this formula:

Emotions = Energy in Motion

And if we don't release that energy, we must work to keep it in. Picture emotions as steam produced in the center of your soul. Steam is a powerful energy source. It can move machines, heat buildings and cook food, but only when guided into the proper channels. If it is capped, the pressure rises to an explosive level — producing a big bang!

Our unexpressed emotions get trapped in our own emotional cookers. Day after day the pressure builds as we keep the lid on our feelings. Then, at some bizarre moment, maybe when the coat hangers won't separate properly, the whole thing blows, emptying in a torrent of emotion.

Allow Yourself to Feel Your Feelings

To prevent emotions from building up these internal barriers, allow yourself to feel whatever feelings are inside you, fighting the desire to judge them as good or bad. Feelings just *are*.

But feelings do not have to control your behavior — or your life. You don't have to withdraw just because you feel rejected. You don't have to scream or wound someone just because you are angry. Nor does it mean you are less godly when you are angry.

The key is to identify and release the feelings in positive ways: writing and lifting them up to God, creating something with your hands, singing, talking or exercising.

Keep a Journal

I found the greatest freedom in learning to express my feelings when I started keeping a journal.

For some time others had encouraged me to keep a journal, but I always protested, "That's not for me!" I didn't think I had the

156

time, the patience — or the privacy. What if someone saw what I had written?

A loving friend helped me look honestly at my protests and asked if they were excuses. Out of respect for her guidance, I began to keep a journal. Taking ten extra minutes of my day, I started on a miraculous journey to a new kind of freedom. In the privacy of my journal's pages, I can say frankly whatever I am feeling.

Remember that my pattern had always been to deal with emotions in the Scarlett O'Hara way: "I don't have time to think about that today. I'll think about it tomorrow." Tomorrow became today when I started journaling. I found that by writing about the daily events in my life, I could touch how I felt about what was occurring. I discovered that under my polite and busy smile were often hurt and anger.

By turning those feelings inward, I was forming a brick wall around my heart — a wall that was separating me from the love, peace and joy I desperately desired. Remember that "a heart at peace gives life to the body" (Proverbs 14:30). I learned not to hide my hurts and frustrations, but rather to acknowledge them and lift them up to God for His healing touch.

Do you feel the same hesitation about journaling that I did? Maybe you think you don't have the time or the privacy. What if your parents or spouse or child discovered it? Or perhaps you hate writing or even thinking about it.

Look again. Are your protests, like mine, excuses? Finding ten extra minutes in a day is a matter of rearranging priorities; getting up a few minutes earlier or ending the busy-ness of your day a little sooner is all you need to do. The enormous release that comes through journaling is well worth the effort. Your self-consciousness will fade, enabling you to write more easily the feelings and thoughts that flood your inner soul and spirit.

Permit yourself to feel the feelings and work through them. This may seem like a journey into unfamiliar and even frightening territory, but journaling can keep you on the path of expressing your feelings. As you journal what you are feeling, you will find unexplainable peace. What is in the light doesn't cause the same degree of uneasiness as what is cloaked in darkness.

✌ Journaling Tips ∾

The journal. I've used both an inexpensive spiral-bound notebook and my portable computer. The journaling vehicle is just the tool.

When to journal. I write nearly every day. Because I look at journaling as a gift of time to myself, I almost feel cheated when I miss a day. I write in the morning at the beginning of my prayer time. Others journal at night before bed, while some people write during any quiet moment in their day.

What to journal. What do I write about? I often start with what has happened to me, but I don't stop there. I write about how I feel about what has happened or what might happen in the future.

You can write about your fears, your inadequacies, your regrets, your joys, your hopes and your discoveries. When you feel happy, write it down. When you feel sad or angry or rejected, tell your journal.

Let your journal help you identify what you are feeling. The act of writing has a way of forcing you to name vague, free-floating feelings. Believe me, there is an enormous power in names. Once you name how you feel about something, you can take power over it. It is no longer an unknown attacker.

As you write about a feeling, you can start to let go of it and process it. When you look at it on paper, you can gain a new perspective about the situation that may have caused the feeling. Why did a certain person or situation trigger such a feeling? Did it remind you of something in your childhood? Did it scratch a memory? Did it make you feel ashamed or inadequate? Is there tension with another person that you need to discuss?

These and similar questions can be answered only in a time of quiet. Your journal can be a tool to help you hear God's call to wholeness, freedom and peace as He leads you "beside still waters" and restores your soul (see Psalm 23:2-3).

The Submerged Emerges

Denial is a formidable and deceptive tool for survival. How easy it is to fill our days and nights with activities so we can ignore and deny our true feelings. How many people do you know who seem to have arranged their lives as I had, so they become "human doings" rather than human beings? A "human doing" is too busy to feel anything.

You may find that just allowing yourself to feel emotions and acknowledge them may be enough to remove some of the logjams to your personal wellness. Whatever the case, don't cling to unhealthy feelings. *What you feel can be healed.* As long as you stuff your feelings with food or cover them up with life's busy-ness, there's no opportunity for healing.

Meeting feelings face-to-face, bringing them out in the open, feeling them and letting them go will renew your mind and give you the space in your heart and the energy for God-given joy, happiness and freedom.

PART THREE

LIVING WELL,
LIVING FREE

THIRTEEN

THE
CHALLENGE
OF CHANGE

I DON'T KNOW what's wrong with me. I love the new way I'm living. I love the way I'm feeling. I love telling about my new life."

These were the words of Katie, whom I described at the beginning. In six weeks she had made some amazing changes in her eating patterns and her perspectives about food. She had lost ten pounds on the scale, and measurements of her muscle-to-fat ratio showed she had lost even more fat. At the same time she was replacing valuable muscle mass that had been lost through years of unhealthy eating and dieting. She looked and felt marvelous, yet clearly something was wrong.

"I started sobbing this morning for no apparent reason," she continued. "I don't know what I'm feeling, but I've been depressed all day. And I blew up in the grocery store yesterday! I couldn't find the cereal I wanted. I just lost it! There were so many cereals to choose from, all claiming to be the best for me, and I just broke down, feeling overwhelmed. It wasn't that I was confused; I knew which to buy. I just don't know what I'm feeling."

I had a clue to what Katie was feeling; it was the challenge of change. Strange as it may sound, I believed she was grieving and thereby experiencing a myriad of emotions from a myriad of sources. As thrilled as she was with the changes in her life, she was sad and mad, panicked and helpless all at the same time. And she was in trouble — her new way of living was under attack.

Katie was grieving over several losses: the carefree, careless way she used to eat; the way she had *used* eating; the foods she always loved; even the weight she was losing for the last time. And that meant change — to a whole new way of eating.

Most of us know that positive life changes don't come easily. A battle rages during the process of taking hold of the new while giving up — yet still hanging on to — the old and familiar. To win this battle, change must come from the inside out, starting with acknowledging the problem and ending with the problem-solver, God.

Pinpoint the Need

The first and biggest step in the challenge of change is to recognize the need for change and passionately desire to bring it about. This desire is critical, since change is hard to face and even harder to carry through. It stirs up old fears within us and can be terrifying. We can remain stuck in old patterns simply because of fear. If we feel stressed and out of control, or the fear is too strong, we are afraid to change.

163

Change is not all bad. Even when prompted by a crisis, change is natural and necessary in life — to keep us moving and growing.

In fact, it was this challenge of change that prompted me to write *The Food Trap*. I had discovered that a lot of people needed more than education to follow through and maintain lasting change; their eating problems seemed to be bigger than the nutritional needs of their bodies. They wanted to eat differently, think about food differently and certainly weigh a different amount, but they could not succeed in those goals. Resistance to change, and the fear of it, seemed to be the glue that kept them stuck.

The Stages of Change

There are five often-difficult stages we must go through before we fully embrace any change.

1. Looking fear in the face

Acknowledging that fear is a natural response to change is important. Denying the threat of the new will only keep you stuck in the old. A wise person once said that we change when the misery of where we are is greater than the fear of change.

Often it's a crisis that gives the wake-up call — telling you that you have to change or else. It may be a doctor telling you to change your eating habits or else go on insulin because of recently diagnosed diabetes. It may be an expensive suit that no longer fits, screaming at you to get in shape. It may be that you're sick and tired — literally. The desire to change must rise up to face the fear.

Most people face five major fears in the process of change:

Fear of the unknown. We are most at ease when we are completely familiar with our surroundings and sure of what the future holds for us. As a result, fear of the unknown can paralyze us.

Strangely, a life filled with constant tragedy may be comfortable and "safe" to us because it's all we've ever known, whereas a life filled with calm may be a frightening prospect.

We all know people whose lives are like soap operas. You meet them on the street and ask, "How are you?" You find out that their electricity was just turned off, they are facing a horrible surgery, their car just blew up, and they just lost their new job. Whenever life threatens to go smoothly, the fear of the unknown pops up and says, "Hey, this is scary. This can't be right!" Very soon another tragedy emerges, and everything returns to "normal."

Fear of failure. People often ask me: "What if I try this new way of eating and don't stick with it? Won't I be a laughingstock?" They expect to do everything right the first time, instead of taking time to work things out and do them right at *some* time.

Some of us see setbacks as valuable learning experiences, while others see setbacks as failures. The fear of failing is a powerful force in the resistance to change.

Fear of commitment. Some people don't set firm goals or accomplish what they set out to do because they fear commitment. They manage to keep postponing what they might like to do with their lives. By setting a goal, they think they will have to accomplish it. When a goal is accomplished, they believe they will have to hold on to it.

They are unsure if a particular goal is the perfect one for them, and they fear getting trapped in the wrong thing. What if something better comes along? What if they choose a goal (such as going back to school or changing their eating patterns) and it turns out to be the wrong decision — and doesn't make them happy?

We need to be honest with ourselves and commit to a few simple, heartfelt goals — what we really dream of doing. Even if it turns out to be less than perfect, we have learned a lot in the process.

Fear of disapproval. Some might consider this to be the fear of rejection. I am frequently asked: "What if I commit myself to my goals and people disapprove?"

When we make positive changes, friends and family often say, "I liked you better the way you were!" Psychologists call this "changeback pressure" from those who feel threatened by your changes. They put subtle pressure on you to change back to the old ways. Expect *someone* to disapprove of your success; it will help you stay successful if you don't expect everyone to be thrilled.

Fear of success. Clients have asked me: "What if I'm successful? Are people going to dislike me or feel uncomfortable around me?" When we make it through some of the changes and are feeling good, we may even feel guilty for feeling good! This can be traced back to our being taught as children that we are selfish for taking care of ourselves. Or it may come from a deep core of shame inside that tells us we don't deserve to succeed.

These fears are not only the obstacles to change, but they are also the very vacuum that sucks us back to the old destructive behaviors. They serve as fuel for setbacks and for sabotage. (For insight into overcoming these fears, see chapters 14 and 15.)

Fear may be a natural feeling, but the natural loses its power in the light of the supernatural, transforming power of God. A first step to releasing the fear comes through choosing to look to God for His power, the same power that raised Jesus to life. He went to the cross and arose from the grave so that you and I could have victory through His redeeming grace.

I love Zig Ziglar's declaration, "Courage is not the absence of fear; it is going on in spite of the fear." And an exciting thing occurs when we do go on. We may find that once we decide to face a fear, it evaporates. How often have you avoided doing a task that you thought would be impossible or particularly embarrassing? When you finally did it, it wasn't half as bad as you anticipated. This particularly applies to owning up to mistakes or misdeeds (such as the time when I had to tell my husband that I had side-swiped the neighbor's mailbox and the side-view mirror — and scraped a good deal of paint off our new car). Thinking about it is much more painful than doing it.

2. Hard work

Most people actually enjoy this stage. It often involves hard mental work. We may take classes, read books and gather information about the subject of our desired change. There's a sense of control in this stage — of working hard to figure out the solution to the crisis.

3. Tough decision

Then we reach the point where we must make a difficult decision — the decision to "just do it!"

4. Unexpected pain

This was exactly where Katie was in the challenge of change. She was doing the right things, but getting the wrong results. Instead of getting easier, change was getting harder. She was expecting to feel wonderful but was actually feeling awful.

Whenever we let go of the old, we experience loss. It happens when we leave a neighborhood we know and love; when we change jobs; when parents die; when children leave the nest. We also experience loss when we let go of old behaviors and habits. In every transition, happy or sad, we're called to let go of what was. Until we do, we can't appreciate what is.

In the case of Katie's lifestyle changes, she hated the way she used to eat but had eaten that way a long time. It was familiar to her. She loved the new foods and patterns of eating but had to let go of the old and the familiar, which she was glad to give up. But she still had to get beyond her grief. The apostle Paul encouraged us to do what he did: "Forgetting what is behind and straining toward what is ahead, I press on toward the goal to win the prize" (Philippians 3:13-14).

In this stage we can't see the positive results of the changes we've made yet, but we do feel the pain of loss. We don't *feel* successful even when success may be right around the corner.

Most of us quit at this point. We don't recognize that the resentment that sets in and the depression, rejection and anger we feel are all part of the grieving process.

Genuine change occurs when we let go of the old and put all our efforts into moving into our new and better patterns of living. As we do, the pain of loss will be balanced by the joy of change.

Keeping a journal will help you identify what otherwise might be vague feelings of anxiety. If you see the frustrations as logjams to your personal wellness and find the strength to go forward from where you've stopped, you will reach the next stage.

It's easy in this stage to rely on your own strength or willpower to change your life. Instead, trust God to be your source of strength. As you embark on your journey to freedom and wellness, you must daily renew your commitment to do it God's way. Come to Him, seek His ways and ask for His guidance. He will comfort, encourage and strengthen you.

5. Joy and transformation

In this stage the changes have become part of your life. You have changed!

Let's look ahead in the next chapter at ways to overcome obstacles in our path to wellness.

FOURTEEN

OVERCOMING SETBACKS

A S YOU EMBARK on any healthy lifestyle change, your body needs time to adjust physiologically and emotionally. It will take at least five to six days before the change begins to feel comfortable physically. You can expect the following:

First and second days: You feel slightly sluggish, irritable and dissatisfied with your eating.

Third day: This will be one of your most difficult days as your body begins to feel the chemical change. It may seem that every cell in your body is crying out for food, particularly something sweet. Expect this day to be a struggle, but not impossible to overcome.

Fourth day: If you make it through the third day without overeating, this one won't be so difficult.

Fifth day: This is the day of the ravenous appetite, you can expect to be hungry for food — not sweets necessarily, just food. You can eat a meal and still think: That was a good appetizer. What else is there to eat?

Sixth and seventh days: By now it is getting easier and easier; you have more energy, and you have more control over your appetite. You are on the road to a lifetime of good eating.

Remember that the third and fifth days are always the most difficult. Circle them on your calendar in red!

I know this may sound more like withdrawal from an addictive drug than simply allowing your body to adjust to a wonderfully healthy way of eating. But let's face reality: Putting *in* healthy foods means leaving *out* the unhealthy, and that means a chemical change — a withdrawal of sorts. You need to know what to expect.

It goes like this: Every Monday morning begins the same. We awaken filled with motivation to get back on the diet, start a new one or just eat better. The 3:30 P.M. arsenic hour arrives, and we fall into forbidden food. Even if we could make it through Monday with a firm resolve, that too would crumble when the withdrawal pains of the third day (in this case, Wednesday) begin. By the time Friday's hungries hit, we know the weekend is here, so why get started again until Monday?

We repeat this pattern week after week. It's a pretty classic pattern and a culprit for many false-start attempts at dieting — part of the reason why so many end in defeat before the first week ends.

If you recognize that the chemical changes are a necessary, but temporary, part of new eating patterns, it will be easier for you to break through into a lifetime of good eating. You will have the strength to speak back to the appetite and hunger and choose instead to eat nourishing, healthy foods.

By the sixth day your energy and appetite will begin to stabilize, and the surprise of feeling good will make it all worth the effort.

Taming the Cookie Monster

Even after you have adjusted physically to a new way of eating and looking at food, you will sometimes crave foods you used to love. It is not uncommon to miss that old favorite. These cravings can be the undoing of your new lifestyle, but not your health. Good health can never be affected by one hot fudge sundae, one piece of birthday cake or one hotdog at a ballgame. It's what giving in to the cravings does to our resolve that can hurt us. We read it as a lapse, which weakens us for a relapse, which sets us up for a collapse, which is the I've-blown-it-now syndrome in a nutshell.

The sooner you realize there is no atonement for a poorly chosen meal, the better off you'll be. Don't try to fast the next day, punish yourself with restrictive dieting or take a laxative. Just choose to get back on track with your nutritious, healthy eating.

You can do this by listening to your body and noting how bad you feel after you've eaten foods that are not good for you. And try to prevent cravings before they strike. Resist getting off track and returning to sporadic, erratic eating. This is especially important when you are the most stressed and most vulnerable to the emotional messages that signal you to eat. When the feelings get too hot to handle, it may seem simpler to return to the old way of eating than to change your way of dealing with life.

Your body has been designed so wonderfully that it will reinforce your choice to eat in a healthier style. Remember the reason why you are avoiding high-fat and sugar-laden foods: They are wellness-robbers. No food is worth the distress, abdominal bloating and sluggishness you can expect after you eat in a less-than-healthy way.

You will walk through vulnerable times — the daily cares of this life, fatigue, personal obligations, holidays — that seem to draw you back to old, predictable patterns. Overcoming each difficult time will make the next one easier.

Among those experiences can be parties, which appear to be quicksand for good intentions. Here are some tips you may find helpful to pull you through those times.

ᴗ: Party Tips for Moderation :ᴗ

- Always eat a healthy snack before going to parties, office celebrations, open houses and the like so you can maintain control over your "appetite for the appetizers." You can choose what, and if, you will taste when you don't arrive famished.

- Never starve yourself on the day of a big party or meal. You will only throw off your metabolism and set yourself up for disaster. Instead, maintain your small, evenly spaced meals throughout the day, which will keep your metabolism and appetite in better control.

- Never tell people you are dieting; it is self-sabotage. You will quickly be talked into eating everything. If you feel you must say anything, just say, "No, thank you." Don't look pitiful and sit in a corner. (No one ever notices that the life of the party isn't eating.)

- Remember that the problem is not the big parties or special events but your day-to-day eating. Avoid the I've-blown-it-now syndrome.

Eating well is a lot like learning to ride a bike; it takes patience, consistency and endurance. If you fall off, so what? It's no problem to climb back on.

Here is the secret to overcoming setbacks: No matter how often you fall off, don't lose heart. The more often you try, the better you'll get. Some days will work out as you have planned, and some won't. And, like bike riding, once you learn to live more healthfully, you'll never forget how good you felt eating right.

FIFTEEN

OVERCOMING SABOTAGE

A MAJOR CHALLENGE in your personal change will be dealing with the reactions of your family and friends. Your change may be as scary to them as it is to you. They are losing a familiar you and getting to know a new you. Often they like the old you a little better, particularly if the old you met their needs — even at the expense of your own.

Many of us are so focused on caring for others that we tend to put our own needs on the back burner. Is it because we get more strokes when we are performing for others than we do when we take care of ourselves? The lack of self-care may be based on the lie that we are not worth taking care of.

As you see yourself in a new light, your image of yourself will not depend as much on how others see you — or their response to you.

Many family members want to see weight loss and success as long as they can control it. If they can take the credit, they will help. But if they think you are doing this on your own, they may decide that they have more to lose than to gain. As unhealthy as you may be in your present state, it may be comfortable for them to have you this way. This is especially true of spouses. Let's look at how husbands, and then wives, can sabotage a mate's efforts. Here are some typical "motivators":

"I'll pay you ten dollars for every pound you lose."

"Lose twenty-five pounds in the next two months, and I'll buy you a new wardrobe."

"Get into that bathing suit, and we'll go on a cruise."

Husbands often try to motivate their wives to lose weight. But, actually, they are the least likely to be helpful since they are too personally involved and too invested in success.

Most often husbands want to see their wives lose weight, but they fall short of offering positive assistance. Why? Subconsciously they may fear their wives' success, and the fear may sabotage any helpful efforts. There is so much at stake: Loss of eating as a form of entertainment and a change of diet may mean that new foods are served while old ones lose their favored-food status. Plus, as a wife becomes more physically attractive, her husband may grow more insecure.

The sabotage may be subtle complaints about the "new way of eating." ("Why don't we ever have anything good to eat anymore?" "This tastes awful! You used to be such a good cook!" "Well, honey, you can eat any way you want, but don't mess with my food. I'm not the one with the problem.")

Sometimes the sabotage is much more direct: He brings home ice cream or doughnuts or boxes of candy.

Katie had been fighting submerged sabotage for her entire married life. Although her husband, Roger, would promise her exotic vacations and wardrobes if she would just "lose this weight," the sabotage would start a few weeks after the diet was showing success. It was very subtle.

Roger would make discouraging remarks, such as "You don't seem to be losing as you should. Are you sure you're not cheating?" or "Are you sure that's on your diet?" or "When is this diet really going to work so I can have a pretty wife again?"

A few weeks later he would bring home "surprises" of Katie's favorite eclairs because she had been so good on that awful diet. Before long he was complaining to friends about how boring and tasteless her cooking had become, and he had to eat out to get a decent meal. All the while he was holding out the promise of that new wardrobe or cruise.

Likewise, wives often sabotage their husbands' attempts to change eating patterns. They start out being supportive: buying and cooking food in a healthier fashion. But when the husband shows signs of succeeding in his health goals (slimming down, gaining energy, keeping an exercise regimen), things change on the homefront.

"Pam, you can't believe it! I came home last night, and Mary had baked macadamia nut, chocolate chip cookies — just for me! She said that I had lost all the weight I needed to lose and that I deserved a special treat. When I tried to say 'thanks but no thanks,' she blew up at me and told me she was sick of all this healthy eating, and it was time things got back to normal."

Ron knew that things weren't going back to the way they used to be. He had embraced a new perspective about wellness that went far beyond his weight — one that he was not about to give up.

Interestingly, Mary had changed right along with Ron and honestly loved their new way of eating and thinking about food. But she didn't expect him to get so attractive again. She didn't feel as secure in their relationship, and she resented Ron's jokingly saying, "Mary was killing me with food!"

Mary's sabotage was a direct result of the fear she was experiencing, similar to Katie's sabotaging husband, but with an added twist: Ron's success seemed to threaten Mary's identity as the provider of "good food." It pinpointed her previous food-buying and cooking patterns as the culprit. If she could sabotage the new patterns and get things back to normal, she could reduce her anxiety.

How can you hold your own against a spouse or others who may not even know he or she is sabotaging your efforts? Anticipate and prepare for other people's reactions. If you can expect others' negative actions and comments, you can minimize their negative effect on you.

Katie held her own by preparing herself for Roger's comments and actions. We planned ways she could respond lovingly to Roger rather than reacting by eating to spite him. She approached this as a way of eating for the whole family, not as her "problem."

Katie was writing in a journal every day, and through her writing she was able to define how she felt, then talk to Roger about it. They began counseling with a pastor from their church to learn to communicate lovingly. Most important, Katie made a decision that she was changing her eating for herself — not to get a new wardrobe or to go on a vacation. Gaining freedom was reward enough.

The only person capable of gaining the freedom you desire for yourself is you. Another person may not force you to change or prevent you from doing so. Another person's words and actions may have an effect on you, but ultimately it is you who decide your actions. You decide what will and won't go in your mouth.

Just Say No!

"Just say no" has been a powerful campaign slogan warning children and teens against drug use. The irony of such a campaign is that we adults can't even say no to a chocolate chip cookie. How can we expect our children to say no to drugs? Peer pressure didn't die in high school. No matter what your age, you must learn — or remember — to say one simple word that tends to get stuck in the human throat: No.

I have my patients practice saying no to the rearview mirror while driving and to the bathroom mirror while shaving or apply-ing their makeup. Just practicing the word and seeing it form on their lips prepares them to "just say no" to unhealthy choices.

When you're offered a food that doesn't fit into your wellness plan, there's no need to give reasons for your action. Neither is there a need to feel guilty, especially when the person offering the food is someone who knows what efforts you are making to change. A caring friend will respect your desire for freedom and will understand a simple "No, thank you."

Of course, not every host (or family cook) is a supportive voice. You will hear discouraging and tempting comments: "Come on — you can splurge tonight. You deserve a little fun once in a while!" "Oh, just a little bit won't hurt." Even, "I think you're carrying this too far. You're in bondage to this nutrition thing."

Again, try to prepare yourself for people's negative responses to the change in your life. Feeding someone rich and "special" foods is often considered a way of expressing love to that person. As you show that you do not equate food with love, such cooks are likely to learn to express their love to you in alternate ways. Answer with a simple "No, thank you." It is your life and your choice for a life of freedom. Self-control is not bondage.

Never say, "I can't eat this." Instead say, "I don't care for any — thank you." Those words communicate strength and decisiveness *and* make a positive confession. The truth is that you *can* eat anything; there are just some foods that you choose not to eat.

Breaking the Power of the Scale

Another agent of sabotage is the scale. For years we have used the scale as a "god" to tell us if we've been good or bad, if we should be happy or sad, if we can eat — or must starve — today. The answers to these questions can never come from a machine that displays a deceptive number that can never, never give the whole truth.

The scale has no indicator that shows how much of your weight is muscle mass, water weight or fat; it just shows a number! That's why we can gain five pounds and think it's "just water weight" and lose five pounds and think it's fat. But the scale can't tell you this kind of information.

If you've been a dieter, the scale may have been your license to eat. You've checked in with the scale to get quick reinforcement for your self-denial. The logic goes like this: If I'm going to give up everything I enjoy in life (my favorite foods), I surely better get some payoff! If the scale doesn't give that reward, I yell, "Not fair! If I'm not going to lose, I might as well be eating." If the scale does show a weight loss, I feel the need to celebrate how good I've been, and, of course, I celebrate with food. Then I weigh myself after the celebration; if I didn't gain, I feel as if I got away with it, which sets me up to try to get away with it again.

But the scale is a lying, deceptive, false god. Weighing every morning or three times a day is part of an obsession with weight and food.

A healthy relationship with food, eating and our bodies is not a matter of how many pounds we weigh on any scale. If we have weight to lose, it should come off as a benefit of being freed from unhealthy eating behaviors and wrong perspectives about food.

This may sound drastic, but it's important. Weigh yourself right now, then don't weigh yourself again for a month. Trust in the healthy way you know you're now eating; trust in how you feel your body changing — not in what a scale is reading.

You may find that giving up this reliance on the scale is more difficult than giving up overeating. Give it a try!

This idea may make you feel threatened, even angry. Many of us rely on the scale as if its "words" were God's. Of course, the scale in itself is not evil. But when we rely too much on those numbers, giving the scale more power than a mechanical device should have, we rob ourselves of any peace we could have.

You may want to close this book for a while and spend a few days observing your eating — and how your body responds. Does the scale have a magnetic power, pulling you toward it for answers? Then come back to these pages. Has your perspective changed? Do you see that the scale indeed holds unhealthy power over your life? Can you trust in God rather than the scale god?

Overcoming Self-Sabotage

"I know the enemy, and he is me." Who said that? I'm not sure of the source, but I am sure of the truth of it. So often we are our deadliest enemy in making positive change. And that, as we already discovered, includes our fears.

An obstacle in the path of change, fear prevents us from succeeding. Some of us won't allow ourselves to succeed in trimming down to an attractive size because of the fear of being a target sexually or of not holding on to the success. The fear is often nothing more than the tip of the iceberg of shame — inner shame that becomes the sabotage of our efforts.

Inner shame becomes a distorter of one's identity. It does not allow someone to say, "I made a mistake." Instead it shouts, "I *am* a mistake! I was born a mistake!"

Inner shame damages our ability to value ourselves. Even with a deep faith in God you can still believe you are somehow "different" and less valuable than others.

This kind of shame is based on what has been said and done to us, often at a very young age. We may not know exactly why, yet we believe it is harder for God to love us than it is for Him to love others. We certainly aren't worth taking care of or loving.

Distorting shame can creep into any kind of family or life situation, not just abusive ones. These are some of the causes:

Words can cause shame. They become tapes that play over and over in your mind. If you hear and believe words that are not true, they can lead you down a destructive path.

Words contain tremendous power. Proverbial wisdom tells us that death and life are in spoken words: "The tongue has the power of life and death" (Proverbs 18:21). As the childhood saying goes, "Sticks and stones may break my bones," but Solomon knew that words *can* hurt me, even to the point of death — killing the truth of who we have been created to be.

Destructive spoken words may include: "You can't do anything right." "You'll never be anything but trouble." "You'll never amount to anything." "If you really love us, you'll make us proud of you." "You're going to fight being fat all your life." "You're so lazy...so unlovable...so dumb...so stupid...such a pig." Such horrible, shaming words, many times spoken carelessly, can control our lives if we let them.

Shaming words are often spoken by people with a high level of inner shame themselves as they try to shift their personal shame onto others.

Abandonment can cause shame. This might be the physical abandonment that comes through divorce, desertion or even death of a parent. Or it could be emotional abandonment; a physically present parent can ignore a child's emotional needs. The adult child can then spend a lifetime trying to fill those unmet needs.

An abandoned child cannot understand why he or she has been deserted or ignored by this all-perfect parent (a child cannot picture a parent as anything less than perfect), so the child bears the responsibility for the wrongdoing, internalizing the shame built on a lie: I must be bad because I made him or her leave me.

Emotional or physical abuse can cause shame. The statistics are staggering. One out of four women has been sexually abused. One out of eight men has been abused.[1]

When the very person who is there to take care of you abuses you, you have been abandoned. The sense of distorting shame is deep, built on a modified version of the lie above: I must be bad, very bad, because I made him or her hurt me.

Some people cannot remember many details of their childhood. In blocking out the intense pain of abuse, they have blocked out the whole time period. Yet the bad days are still there, locked in the subconscious, creating shame, false guilt and a horrible distortion of self-worth.

This distorting shame can rob you of your identity. If you think you are a mistake or a second-class citizen, the opinions of others become more important than your own. Their opinions of you become your sole measure of who you are. Even success cannot overcome this shame. The shame tells you that you don't deserve success or good things. You may fear that others will find out about the "real you." Because of the shame, you may work to undermine any success that comes your way.

Shamed people tend to be frustrated and angry in their powerlessness against other people because they think others are more important than they are.

Covering Shame

What can fill or cover our shame? We look for a temporary balm to soothe our shame — or our feelings of loneliness and abandonment. Addictions or mood-altering experiences can be momentary soothers. But the bad feeling doesn't go away; the hole inside isn't filled easily, so we keep going back for more. We may choose alcohol, drugs, relationships to fill the vacuum — or the more acceptable vice: food.

When we are in shame, not believing our needs count, we cover up our needs. If we depend on food to satisfy our emotional needs, at some point in childhood we probably began meeting our legitimate emotional needs in this illegitimate way — with food.

Most adults with eating dependencies started out overeating in response to stress. As children we depended on food to protect us from pain that we had no power to remove. As adults we continued overeating to deny our feelings and to block the intimacy of close relationships.

Compulsive overeating is one coping skill that can numb the pain. Denying oneself food by dieting or starving through the day may be a means of trying to take control of the pain.

As our lives become more complicated and stressful, the demand for food increases. It becomes a life preserver in the midst of the storm — something to hang on to for life. And trying *not* to eat isn't the answer; it represents drowning in the pain and must be avoided.

Are You Feeling Stuck?

I mentioned earlier that this challenge of change had prompted me to write *The Food Trap*. I had discovered a group of clients who seemed hopeless and helpless — unable to make long-lasting, positive changes.

These clients seemed to depend on food and eating in such a way that they required a type of counseling far beyond nutritional helps. Even after seeing some change, they would actually be almost sucked back into their old ways. With each attempt they became more disillusioned and desperate; they had no idea why they weren't getting free from food and diets.

If you feel discouraged and confused and not at all free; if you are struggling to maintain a positive eating change, it's time to look further. I want to tell you what I tell my clients as they hit walls in working out their freedom. I want you to have more insight on eating changes and take a deeper look at the food trap.

It may be time to look to the emotional you and evaluate your relationship with food and your body. Are you eating to deal with what's eating you? Are you using food to cope with life? Are you meeting your emotional needs through the use — and abuse — of food and eating?

PART FOUR

THE
FOOD TRAP

HEALTHY
BELIEFS

TWO MONTHS AFTER her initial visit to me, Katie had made many changes. For the first time in her life she was eating in a more balanced way, and she desired foods that would benefit, not harm, her body. Katie had even started walking most afternoons as a powerful stress release. And, amazingly, she had lost thirteen pounds of fat — not muscle or water, and not by starving. It was all a result of her change in eating.

Yet Katie was seeing a new side to her eating habits. "I can do really well on a diet for a while, but then a birthday or a holiday comes up, and I just have to eat something really 'good.' I can give up everything I love — chocolate, cookies, chips — for a while, but I can't imagine life without them. I'm really enjoying new foods, prepared new ways, but how could I enjoy life without the old foods I love?"

Katie realized that if she was eating the right things at the right time she was not as likely to overeat or to eat poorly — even though she wanted to in response to every emotion, especially stressful ones. Katie was most desirous of the old "favorites" when she felt hurt or rejected. Then she felt she could not control the desire; it seemed to control her. All it took was a holiday — or a particularly stressful day — to prompt a binge of the foods she "loved."

Yet Katie was coming to understand that "loving" food was about much more than taste buds. In reality she had an emotional relationship with food that had started years earlier. When she was a child, Katie had discovered that eating certain foods made her feel better — and eating a lot of certain foods made her feel a lot better!

To make permanent changes that would stand up under stress, she had to uncover and look at the roots of her unhealthy relationship with food. Katie had grown up in a very chaotic family, and she had learned early in life to use food to dull her senses and relieve stress. To detach emotionally from food permanently, she had to break her dependence and repair the cracked foundation blocks.

Just Friends

A healthy relationship with food is one of friendship, where food is regarded as the nourishment it was created to be. There is no good or bad food, no legal or cheating food. Food is simply food.

But food is not simply food in the world today. It can be nourishment, but it also can be a source of pleasure. One thing is for sure — it certainly does more than satisfy hunger. Like Katie, many of us grew up eating in response to *every* emotion.

I sure did. As a family we ate to celebrate when we were happy; to feel better when we were sad; to give us something to do when we were bored; or to gain control when we felt frustrated. I ate to stuff down my anger and soothe my nerves. I entered adulthood believing that any problem in life could be solved with a banana split!

Generally, we have been taught that food makes us feel better, and sometimes it does. Most of us use food at one time or another to reduce the tension or pain of the moment, and then we return to a normal way of eating once the uncomfortable feeling has passed.

But some of us do not return to a normal pattern of eating. The logic goes something like this: If food made me feel good yesterday, it should today, and if today, then it will tomorrow too. We can become as dependent on food as we can on any chemical substance, and it can be as destructive as any addiction.

Hooked on Food?

Yes, millions of Americans are hooked — emotionally dependent — on food. What does that mean?

It has nothing to do with your present weight; you may be very overweight or very thin. Rather it has to do with an improper relationship with food in which food and eating have assumed an unnatural importance in your life. They dominate the physical, emotional and spiritual you. In this improper, love-hate relationship, food has an unnatural control over you. You may love the way it tastes and makes you feel, but you hate it for what it does to your body and how it controls your life. Like any unhealthy relationship, it results in a roller coaster of emotions: gratification and satisfaction, guilt and remorse, being "good" only to be "bad." The obsession fills your thoughts and actions, robs you of well-being and affects your self-esteem; it holds you captive. It has life-damaging consequences.

Food is a trap when it is used as a substitute for love, friendship or success, or when it's used to cover up more serious emotional issues. Unhealthy eating and overeating can become a way of life and a way of coping with life. And because we must eat for life, we obviously can't abstain from it as we can from other abusive substances. Food is quite another story, even for people who have given up smoking.

Food is not inherently evil. Humans must have it to survive and thrive; we are physically dependent upon it. God created us to need food, and He created us to enjoy the taste of food. He also designed the eating of it to be pleasurable while we're benefitting from its nourishment.

The problems begin when we become emotionally dependent on food to cope with everyday life, when it becomes our source of joy. Food becomes an evil when we love eating more than we love ourselves, more than we love other people and more than we love God.

People who never touch alcohol, drugs or cigarettes often use food as their vice or real pleasure in life. How many church socials I've attended where people proudly declare they don't need liquor to have a good time — but don't dare take away their cake table!

Scripture is full of illustrations about food and gluttony, messages often ignored. Food — and finances — are two vulnerable issues for us because we can't live without them. Many do well in the abstinence issues; denominations are even formed around them. We find strength in abstinence. We can live without alcohol, nicotine and narcotics — even though withdrawal can be deadly. But food and money are not objects we can abstain from; we must have them to survive.

We must apply the fruit of self-control to them, however, and keep them in their appropriate place — not loving them more than God or more than people. And that's why they become a trap. That's why the Bible calls the love of money the root of all sorts of evil (see 1 Timothy 6:10) — not because it is inherently evil, but because it can so easily become a lord over our lives. Neither is food inherently evil until it becomes our golden calf.

As Scripture records in Exodus 32, God, Moses and the top of Mount Sinai seemed too far away for the Israelites waiting in the valley below. Anxious for a quick-fix god that they could see and touch, the Israelites molded a calf of gold.

We likewise turn to food because it's always at hand and gives immediate gratification.

FOOD FOR LIFE

A Golden Calf or Golden Arches?

How often, when we face difficult circumstances, does God seem too far away? How often do we turn to another "god" (soda, chocolate, ice cream or the golden arches) to make us feel better? How often do we use food to alleviate an uncomfortable situation? Of course, like the golden calf, food is a false god. Our hunger for an all-powerful God can be momentarily quelled by overeating, but it will never be satisfied. Eating can never fulfill us, give us peace or take away the pain. It just adds more stress, because now we have guilt on top of the other emotions!

Although this may sound overly dramatic, it's reality. We are killing ourselves with food — cutting our days on this earth short and robbing the life from the days we *are* here. This food trap ruins a person's health and causes guilt, suffering and anguish.

As Jesus warned, "Be careful, or your hearts will be weighed down with dissipation, drunkenness and the anxieties of life, and that day will close on you unexpectedly like a trap" (Luke 21:34).

Born to Be Free

All of us desire change for our lives — genuine change. We try to commit to making that change, but we simply can't follow through on our commitment. We can make lists of what to do to try to change ourselves, but we remain powerless to break free from destructive patterns.

Identifying the problem is the first step on the road to freedom and change. By naming the problem — whether it is using food to deal with emotions or being too dependent on food to cope with life — you stop denying the problem. You meet it face-to-face. Like a lamp shining in the darkness, your healthy actions illuminate the enemy. No longer is an unknown enemy stalking you without your knowing when, where or how it will strike.

Until you acknowledge the food trap or any trap in which you are ensnared, you will struggle with the belief that you are simply a weak person with no self-control or willpower. Many people suffering from serious eating illnesses spend their lives saying, "I can lose weight; I just have to make up my mind to do it," or "I don't have a problem with food — I just love chocolate!" But it's often a much deeper issue than that.

It is not natural to control eating; it is unrealistic to think that any of us can muster enough willpower to control eating for a lifetime. Remember that the problem in the garden of Eden wasn't the apple; it was the "pair" on the ground.

SEVENTEEN

IS THE REFRIGERATOR LIGHT THE LIGHT OF YOUR LIFE?

W E USE FOOD for purposes it was never meant to fulfill. Let's look at some of our unhealthy — and false — beliefs:

- Food (or dieting) helps us cope with stress, frustration and the insecurities of life. Overeating seems to smooth away the rough edges and relieve the tension, thus allowing us to cope. It provides a quick fix.

- Food (or dieting) fills the gaps in our lives. Food can be a friend and companion who is with us no matter what. When we're lonely, eating seems to fill the emptiness. It substitutes for love, attention and pampering. When we're happy, it's a way to celebrate — even if we're not with other people. When we're working hard with seemingly little recognition or appreciation, food becomes a justly earned reward and comfort.

- Food (or dieting) gives us a sense of identity and control. Loving and controlling food are a lot safer than loving people. When life seems most out of control, rigid denial of food or counting every calorie — even planning a binge — gives a sense of being very much in control of at least one area of life.

- Food (or dieting) helps us sabotage the "perfect image." If we were obedient, people-pleasing children, or if we are that kind of adult, we can use food as a nice way to be bad. Even though becoming overweight is a risk, and often the result, overeating is an acceptable vice and a passive form of rebellion.

- Food (or dieting) helps us deal with deep-seated emotions and feelings. Keeping our minds on food can keep them off the issues of the heart. Overeating is a safe way to express hidden emotions; stuffing food is a way to stuff feelings, to numb them, to shut them off.

The satisfied feeling we get from food fills the gaps — temporarily. But, typically, the more we eat, the more depressed we get, and the more we then eat to feel better. Because food is the quick fix, we never get the chance to fill in the gaps permanently and in healthy ways.

As long as we are eating we do not have to deal with our emotions and pain. If we turn to food every time we get angry or hurt; if we turn to food when an event triggers a painful memory in our past, we never have the opportunity to process the anger or release the pain. Instead we compact pain on top of pain — into a wall around our hearts.

Life at this point can get more and more complicated. Have you ever wondered why so many overweight, overeating people appear to be jolly? Often they are the most angry and the most hurt, but they keep those emotions stuffed. Many, never having been able to express their feelings, become people-pleasers who have little or no way to protect themselves emotionally from demands others place on them. But we need those shields that separate and protect us from others; when all else fails, excess weight can be that shield.

Becoming overweight can also protect someone who is fearful of life from having to deal with certain issues. The reasoning goes like this: If you are overweight, you won't be as attractive to the opposite sex and thereby won't have to risk having relationships and possibly becoming a victim.

As you may recall, I spent the better part of my life thinking about problems "tomorrow." But I needed something to help me push those problems into tomorrow, and food fit the bill. By the time I was in college, food had become my emotional escape-hatch. I didn't have to wait on God if eating could make me feel better; I was emotionally and spiritually dependent upon food. For me, relief was just a swallow away!

I could cover up my eating dependencies with pendulum swings in my weight. I could overcome overeating as long as I was walk-ing in the iron-will discipline of a diet. To cope with emotions, I could replace the obsessive use and intense preoccupation with food with obsessive and intense preoccupation with dieting. The diet would become my fuel. I could focus excessively on dieting and/or an exercise routine and get my weight down. Unfortu-nately, it was short-lived.

As long as we can mask our eating problems with periodic stabs at willpower, we can deny our real problems, believing that a little more discipline, motivation or the right diet would make the real problem go away.

Remember my Orlando-to-Dallas seatmate, Howard? This was exactly where he lived and exactly why any dieting would just be a

Sucrets solution for him. It would reduce the symptoms for a moment but would allow the real problem to rage until treated properly — at the root.

Howard's real problem was what he ate to help him deal with what was eating him. The stress in Howard's job was intense and constant. He appeared to handle it well because he was using food to cope with all the tensions and fears. If he wasn't eating, he was thinking about wanting to eat but knowing he shouldn't. When he was dieting, he would fill his mind with the dieting rules and let those become his focus. But ultimately he would have a lapse. For all his hard work, he would reward himself with a doughnut. That put him into the I've-blown-it-now syndrome, so he would eat a dozen doughnuts.

He would then tell himself, "I've really blown it now, so I'll diet tomorrow."

His eat-today, diet-tomorrow outlook meant that today he ate everything he couldn't have when he dieted tomorrow. It's almost a last-supper mentality. In short, his momentary lapse became a relapse which led ultimately to his collapse.

An eating dependency like Howard's is the result of a lifetime of complex issues. Each person is unique, and each person's situation is different. Some people have extremely painful and debilitating life experiences and have attached their emotions to food. Others don't and may be only mildly affected. Yet a common thread runs through all the experiences; it involves relationships with other people, ourselves and God.

EIGHTEEN

LOOKING
BACK

THEIR STORIES ARE varied, yet time after time I've seen people who have been caught in the food trap at a young age. It was then that they developed a faulty system for covering up emotions and meeting their own needs.

As adults we may appear to be coping with day-to-day life. But all the while, underneath, the child in us is suffering from an overwhelming sense of shame or guilt, self-denial, distrust or too much responsibility — that is, taking on burdens that are not ours to carry.

We have all developed a faulty system in one way or another. It is part of humanity. It is based on the same lie used on Eve in the garden (see Genesis 3:1-6). The lie is this: 1) No one, not even God, can or will meet your needs. 2) You need to be your own god. If you are going to get your needs met, you'd better develop your own system for getting them met. 3) If you get your needs met in an unhealthy way or, as Adam and Eve did, in a sinful way, you won't experience any negative consequences.

As you continue to read about the early family life you may have had, ask which if any patterns have influenced your beliefs and coping mechanisms. If you did not learn as a child how to meet your emotional and spiritual needs properly, you will as an adult be more susceptible to life's traps, including the food trap.

The Family System

Families must have boundaries and rules, and healthy families discuss these rules, listening to each other's opinions. A disagreement about rules wouldn't necessarily mean the rules would change. But in a healthy family, disagreement would be allowed, and all family members would continue to be respected and accepted.

In a healthy family, a child has the opportunity to develop a sense of identity and self-esteem when personal thoughts and feelings are listened to and given value. This child will grow up able to express feelings more freely and openly, with the ability to choose when and where to do so in order to be considerate of others.

But not all of us were raised in healthy families. Some of us were not allowed to voice thoughts and feelings that conflicted with the rules or with our parents. Growing up in these types of families makes it more difficult for us to learn who we are, that our feelings are valid and that we are indeed valuable.

Katie had never learned as a child to own, or certainly value, her feelings. If Katie said she was cold, her mom would say, "You couldn't be. It's burning up in this house." If Katie said she was hungry, her mom would say, "You couldn't be. We just finished lunch." If Katie said she wasn't hungry, her mom would say, "Of course you are. It's dinnertime."

Katie learned early that disagreeing with her mother's I-know-what-you-need-better-than-you-do methods only caused conflict. She came to believe that she was a bad child for even thinking, much less feeling, differently. This grew into a deep sense of shame. She concluded that since her thoughts and her feelings were not valuable, she was not valuable.

The incredible tragedy of unhealthy family systems is that, apart from the grace of God, they are self-propagating. People who have grown up in unhealthy situations often marry each other, and then they raise their children in the same atmosphere of shame. The curse can follow to the third and fourth generations.

Children from these family systems become afraid to express themselves until eventually they don't have a clue as to who they are or how they feel. They learn to avoid conflict at any price, to fear constant rejection and to swallow "unacceptable" thoughts and feelings so they don't upset others.

Was this the case with your own family?

A big part of our healing comes in understanding that our parents were often victims themselves. Many were raised in an atmosphere of shame and grew up not having their own emotional, or even physical, needs met. Unable to meet their own needs, these adults most likely cannot meet the needs of their children. Instead they establish an oppressive set of rules that prevent the healthy expression of feelings. Or they desert their children — physically or emotionally — by placing other things (work, alcohol, golf, even church) above their needs. Or they hurt their children in the same way they were hurt. Tragic situations often yield tragic results: abuse in every form.

Yet most parents did not set out to hurt their children. Many of our parents simply did the best they could with what they had — or knew — to give.

You are not responsible for how you were treated as a child, but you are responsible to take positive steps to do something about it now. Understanding what kind of family system you grew up in will help you break the cycle.

Three Family Types

Eating dependencies most often come out of three types of unhealthy family systems: the perfect family, the overprotective family and the chaotic family. Let's look at these types of families and the messages they send to their members.

The perfect family. This family places a high priority on appearances — the family's reputation, identity and achievements. Its ruling question is, What would people think? Parents in this type of family long to hear people say, "My, don't you have well-behaved children!"

The perfectionistic family does not make mistakes. From the outside looking in, this will seem to be a very loving and caring family. Actually, the loving and caring often cover up a rigid set of rules, many of which govern emotions — especially "weak" emotions. ("Don't cry, or I'll give you something to cry about." "If you can't show a happy face, don't show me a face at all.")

Tapes played in this family are performance-oriented: "A job worth doing is worth doing well." "Make us proud of you." "Don't disappoint us!" "Be good!" "You are my perfect daughter/my perfect son." "Don't ever let us down."

Brigette came from a family like this and turned to food to meet the needs her family failed to meet.

Food was both an enemy and a friend to Brigette — something that both evaded her control and served as a pressure valve for the stress of living a life of perfection. Every binge started the same way: She would feel like, but resist, eating something sweet. The desire would continue to gnaw at her. With guilt fluttering in her conscience, she would run an errand and come home with cookies, frozen yogurt and cheesecake. She would tell herself, just one cookie, maybe two. Definitely not more than four.

After she had eaten the entire bag of cookies, a piece of cheesecake and two big bowls of frozen yogurt, she would sit, stunned, and ask, "Why did I do that?" She would be full, uncomfortably full, with her stomach hurting and bloated. Then, no matter what time of night it was, Brigette would force herself to ride the stationary bike to exhaustion to "work it off," resolving not to do it again.

The overprotective family. This family emphasizes the need to be close — very close. Members tend to take too much responsibility for one another, especially if one has a problem. There are no boundaries in this family; everyone is community property. Slogans of this family include: "All for one and one for all." "You know we'll always be there for you." "You can't trust anyone outside the family." "No one is good enough for you." "Are they 'our' type of people?" "No one can love you the way we do."

Members stay enmeshed within this family because they never develop an independent life of their own. Even as adults they do not evolve unique personalities. Parents in these families work hard to be good, caring parents. They just never quite see and hear their children clearly.

This was the case in Merritt's family. She turned to food because she had no way of gaining attention or getting her needs met in her family. She had to find a way to feel better all by herself, a way to stay afloat in the midst of the storms at home and in her heart. Overeating became Merritt's life preserver — everything her family wasn't.

Food was readily available and something she could get for herself. It never let her down; she could always count on it to make her feel better. Dieting to Merritt meant letting go of her life preserver. Without food she feared she would drown.

The chaotic family. The rules of this family either do not exist or are inconsistent because the parents are unavailable emotionally to their children. Abuse, either physical or emotional, takes place in this family.

A child may be neglected because of alcoholism or workaholism. Some parents may provide ample material things but be emotionally unavailable for or abusive to the children.

The children of chaotic families learn not to talk, trust or feel. Because they deaden their emotions, they do not acknowledge their feelings or their reality.

Like the others, standard tapes play in these families too: "Don't ask questions. Do as you're told." "You can't trust anyone." "Do as I say, not as I do." "Because I said so!" "I wouldn't yell at you if I didn't love you." "This hurts me more than it hurts you."

Dana came from a family like this. For Dana, overeating helped numb the pain of her life. When emotion would start to rise up, whether rejection or anger or fear, food was a way to push it back down. Even the yo-yo dieting she began as a teenager helped to sedate her emotions; while dieting she could keep everything in her head, thinking about facts and figures and trying to be "good," and not deal with the hurt in her heart. As long as she was on The Diet, she could be thinking obsessively about what she couldn't eat or when she could eat next. This kept her from feeling. But once off the diet, Dana returned to food and overeating to fill the void.

All of these families are the result of unhealthy rules that have been passed down from generation to generation; accompanying pain and tragedy have been the curse passed down with them. These are not evil or bad people; they are a group of people being controlled by a set of bad rules with lives built on shame.

When you get to the point where you can make an adult commitment to live your own life and to release the past, your relationship with food will take on a whole new character. But to break free, you have to release the past completely. Identify the problems your childhood upbringing may have caused. But don't get stuck in blaming others for these problems, or the hurt, bitterness and anger will keep you stuck in the problem. Blaming and unforgiveness take on a life of their own and keep you in a victim role.

Some people find it helpful to sit down and analyze the relationships in their childhood family. Look at this as a new kind of family tree, linking relationships. The tool on the next page may enlighten you to the tapes that continue to play within you and the systems in which you may be caught.

∾ A Different Kind of Family Tree ∾

Consider these questions carefully:

1. Look at the relationships in your family, between your mother and dad, grandmother and grandfather, parent and children, sibling and sibling. What dynamics characterized each relationship?

2. Look at significant life events or family landmarks. What light did each shed on the dynamics of relationships?

3. What strengths did you learn from the family systems? From your mother? From your father?

4. What weaknesses or negative character traits did you learn?

5. What were the beliefs and motives of the family system?

6. What did your family teach you about God?

7. Describe your relationship with your parents now (even if they are no longer living).

What systems are making you powerless to break free of the food trap? Allow any new information that surfaces in this family tree to be transformed by the renewing of your mind.

Emotionally Starved Teens

Emotions lie at the heart of many eating problems, especially in adolescence. Teens experience pressure from every direction — from peers, teachers, parents, themselves. As an escape from these strains, many indulge in food. Others eat dangerously little as a way of gaining control.

The two most common eating disorders suffered by teens are anorexia nervosa, characterized by excessive weight loss, and bulimia, characterized by food binges, vomiting and constant craving for food. In both illnesses the teens become oblivious to the natural, internal cues of hunger or satisfaction. Eating or starving gives a charge that fills emotional voids.

Often the problem occurs when a teen perceives parental pressure to excel in academics or sports or any endeavor as a need to be perfect. The parent communicates, or the child perceives that the parent is communicating, "Who or what you are isn't good enough."

Obviously, not all teens with quirky eating habits are clinically ill. But when parents observe some compulsive behavior related to their teen's eating or weight, they should try to find out the cause before the symptoms get out of hand. It may be wise to seek a professional opinion or evaluation.

The essential factor in any eating disorder is the attitude toward food and dieting. But the person with a clinical eating disorder also has a distorted image of his or her body appearance. Emaciated people see themselves as fat, and overweight people see themselves as thinner than they are. These are internal perceptions and have nothing to do with reality. These internal messages fuel the eating relationship.

Estimates about how many people are afflicted with clinical eating disorders vary from researcher to researcher. As many as one out of three college women engages in some kind of binging and purging.[1] Clinical eating disorders are seen in both women *and* men.[2] Victims of the disease go beyond teenagers; I see grandparents, professional athletes, homemakers, students and successful career people who are also affected.

Let's take a closer look at bulimia and anorexia, the two most common clinical eating disorders.

What Is Bulimia?

Bulimia is an extreme obsession with food that is defined by the way in which food is consumed, most often in a frenzied, binging pattern, combined with some sort of purging. Purging may involve extended fasting, vomiting, use of laxatives or intense exercise.

A person who binges takes in large amounts of food in a brief time, and binging means different things to different people. Some bulimics report consuming up to forty thousand calories and taking as many as six hundred laxatives a week. Some binge every day. Some purge after any meal or snack, claiming they feel bloated and fat no matter what they eat.

Many compulsive eaters say they first started to purge in hopes of gaining relief from the guilt and bloatedness of overeating.

Although a food binge seems, and feels, out of control, it is actually all about control. You are safe and secure while binging. Your need for love is being met at a steady pace; your feelings are sedated, and you are totally in control of food. You may be out of control of every other aspect of life; but you buy food, you prepare it and you eat it. That makes you totally in control, not needing anyone else. When you are frightened, you most likely can't think of any way to get relief except through binging.

Anorexia: Frozen Emotions

A person with the eating illness of anorexia also has an obsession with food, but to an opposite extreme. The anorexic has an unnatural *fear* of food and is obsessed with *not* eating. As she deprives herself of food, she sedates herself against feelings, much as she can with binging; not eating can put her into a trancelike state in which she is void of feelings. With anorexia, if she doesn't eat, she doesn't feel.

The anorexic takes the control a step further than the bulimic.

By not eating he or she feels invincibly in control. By not needing food, the anorexic can also be saying that he or she doesn't need *people*. It is a desperate statement of the need for control: I want to protect myself from the need for love.

Sometimes anorexia starts with rigid dieting. Maybe some teasing about getting "chubby" or "plump" fuels a fear of food. Maybe societal pressure to be thin and glamorous is internalized in the extreme. A teenager failing an important test or tryout at school might be flooded with those I'm-out-of-control feelings. How can she gain control in one part of her life? By rigidly dieting. Criticism and concern from others often causes an anorexic's problems to worsen; as she feels rejected, she may withdraw further from people.

Getting Help

I wrote this book to help shine a light on areas of darkness in our physical, emotional and spiritual lives, but *Food for Life* may not be enough for you. If you are dealing with the deep issues of anorexia or bulimia, you will need direct help through professional counseling. Use this book in conjunction with counseling, but don't use it in place of counseling.

Many groups are available to aid eating disorder victims and their families. These groups offer detailed information to victims and refer them to doctors and treatment centers. One such group is the National Association of Anorexia Nervosa and Associated Disorders (ANAD), Box 7, Highland Park, IL 60035; (312) 831-3438.

Please go for help. You *are* worth helping, and you deserve to live well.

NINETEEN

RELEASING
THE
PAST

COMING TO TERMS with our families, our feelings and our past can give a freedom not only from the food trap but from the whole destructive system of behavior associated with it. The way out of the cycle of shame is to meet it face-to-face, to bring it out in the open. It requires trust — in God, in ourselves, in others. But the conditions of our upbringing often keep us from trusting anyone or anything.

Yet our needs are met through relationships. A vital, personal relationship with God and honest relationships with others pave the way to healing. God can use other discerning people to help us see our underlying problems.

We were created with a natural need to be understood and accepted. Nonjudgmental relationships — whether they are with trusted friends, a counseling support group, a small home-care group or a ministry team — show wounded people that they can trust again. They reflect God's love for us and can meet needs for intimacy and build up our self-esteem in ways that our family may never have been able to.

The apostle Paul admonishes Christians to "carry each other's burdens" (Galatians 6:2). In another epistle in which he writes about the unity of the church, he says to speak "the truth in love" so that we might grow and be built up in love, "as each part does its work" (Ephesians 4:15-16).

Take a Risk

As you reach out for freedom, I encourage you to take another great leap of faith: Acknowledge your emotional dependency on food to at least one other human being. Choose this confidant carefully and prayerfully — perhaps a trusted friend, a counselor at your church or a professional therapist. I encourage my patients who are dealing with issues such as sexual abuse, incest or alcohol in the family to seek professional counseling and therapy. These are deeply painful issues that affect every part of your being. A professional counselor has the skills to help you walk through — and out of — painful memories.

Not everyone needs a professional counselor, but a person with whom you can share your secret is very important. When you are ready to come out of hiding and go for help you are saying, "I am worth helping."

Human support is vital to breaking free from the food trap. But while others can care, they cannot fix. As food is not your ultimate comforter, neither are people your ultimate source of health and well-being. People will never be able to anticipate your needs as quickly as you'd like. No one is at your side twenty-four hours a day.

The psalmist David knew this when he said, "Though my father and mother forsake me, the Lord will receive me" (Psalm 27:10). He's the same writer who penned the promise of comfort: "The Lord is my shepherd; I shall not want...He restores my soul" (Psalm 23:1,3, NKJV). In the words of the apostle Paul, that would translate, "He renews my mind!" (see Romans 12:1-2).

Choose Forgiveness

You can never go back and relive your early life. But God can restore what has been robbed from you and use for your good what may have been meant for evil.

Have you ever dropped a glass, shattering it into little pieces? Our lives are very much like those broken fragments.

Now picture a beautiful stained glass window — a marvelous work of art made of pieces of broken glass, yet new and complete. With God's healing and restoration you can walk in a new reality made from those shattered pieces.

Two major problems, however, can prevent us from being renewed and restored: not forgiving and not receiving forgiveness. Accumulated unforgiveness, like those bricks we've discussed, adds up, and it weights us down. Those bricks of unforgiveness can also become a wall that separates us from God, others and freedom.

As you look at your past, you will experience emotions that need to be lifted up for processing and healing. God wants to reach into that child's heart inside you and lift your burdens. But you must, through journaling or prayer, be totally honest, identifying and sharing the hurts — all the hurts — you feel.

In the beatitudes Jesus said, "Blessed are those who mourn" (Matthew 5:4). By getting in touch with your pain over what was and what was not in your past, and by releasing and grieving for that pain, you can gain a sense of closure to that part of your life. What happened to you broke your heart and the heart of God. Grieve for that. Say good-bye to your childhood — and grieve for that loss. Those who grieve well, live well as they walk into abundant life. Remember that we have to let go of the old to embrace the new.

Many people write a private letter to their primary caretaker in childhood. They never mail the letter, but in it they express the hurts they experienced as a child. They identify in writing their emotional or physical needs that were not met. Such a letter can help you grieve for what you wanted and needed but didn't receive. One client, encouraged by her therapist to write such a letter, shared it with me and gave me permission to share it with you:

Dear Mommy and Daddy,
My counselor asked me to write you and tell you what I wanted and needed most from you, but you could never give me.
Daddy, I needed you to be there for me. I don't mean just at home; you were there, in body, every night. But I don't ever remember you even talking to me or hugging me or really noticing me unless I had done something bad that day. You were always so mad and tired. I needed you to look at me. I needed to know that I was lovable. I needed to know that *you* loved me.
Mommy, you were always so faithful to provide me with everything I needed: You washed and ironed my clothes; the house was always spotless; you cooked wonderful food for us. But I needed you to listen to me. I needed you to care about how I felt, not just what I should do. I needed you to say you loved me. I needed you to show you loved me.
I know that all of these needs are still there because it hurts so much to write this letter to you. But I am asking the Lord to heal these hurts. I can never be your little girl again to get these needs met. I need to grow up now.

I love you,

Your daughter

Once the hurts are on paper, release the people who were the vehicles for those hurts. Release them to God, who wraps His loving purposes around our hearts and changes us.

I love the Old Testament story of Joseph. Now there was a man who had reason to resent, even hate, his brothers, who had sold him off as a slave. Years later, when Joseph met them face-to-face, he was given the grace to see God's redemptive perspective on the situation. Speaking to his brothers, Joseph said, "You intended to harm me, but God intended it for good to accomplish what is now being done" (Genesis 50:20). Joseph did not hold on to any bitterness against his family, nor did he blame God for painful experiences, which included years in prison.

Forgiveness does not come freely or naturally. Releasing bitterness, especially when it seems justifiable and attached to painful experiences, requires a choice, and it requires the grace of God. As justified as it may seem to blame the things of our past, we must see it as just that, the past. To move on, we need to take our eyes off the problem and who or what may have caused it and focus on living a life filled with freedom, peace and joy.

Freedom for Katie, Freedom for Us

Katie began to break free of the food trap when she started identifying the unhealthy emotional and spiritual seeds that had been sown in her life.

Her family life had planted seeds of low self-worth that determined how she lived her life. Because she had never attached value to her thoughts and feelings, she had no reason to treat her body as anything other than an object to be scorned. As a child Katie learned to love food because it made her feel better. As a teen she learned to hate it because it made her fat. But as she noticed that eating didn't make everyone fat, she concluded she must be as defective as she had always thought she was.

Katie's relationship with God reflected her relationship with her parents. She felt she could get God to love her only if she did good things and didn't make trouble. She didn't always love herself, so why should God love her?

As Katie named the unmet needs of her childhood and grieved for them, her emotional vacuum started filling up with God's love for her. She stopped blaming God for making her the way He had. She began to embrace God's perspective of her — a treasure, a precious child.

Walking in freedom for Katie meant eating in a way that met her needs physically — so that she could let her new relationships with God, herself and others meet her spiritual and emotional needs. Food was no longer to be the protective barrier between Katie and the world, Katie and God. "My eyes are ever on the Lord, for only he will release my feet from the snare" (Psalm 25:15).

The Power Exchange

We have been designed and destined for a lifestyle of freedom. The Revolutionary War patriot Patrick Henry expressed this in a passionate battle cry: "Give me liberty or give me death!"

Yet, no matter what popular thought may say, we are not born free; we are born to *be* free. Spiritual freedom comes with knowing God and His desires for our lives.

It breaks His heart when He sees us ensnared in the traps of the world. He knows that if we are caught in struggles over food, we are not free to work on our heart issues. We are not free to love God — and others — as we love ourselves.

As you embark on your journey to freedom and wellness, you must renew your commitment each day to living free. Take a daily diversion. My life, like yours, is so full of demands that I must have regular, replenishing investments from God. I require quietness to hear the gentle voice of God, to seek His ways and ask His guidance. In the quiet times He comforts and encourages me.

Again, information does not change lives; revelation does. Grasp hold of one truth and let it take root in you and change your life. Each day, every moment of the day, we have voices within casting a vote over us. The enemy of life casts a vote of hopelessness and unworthiness. That voice says, "You can never change. Look at the life you've had, what you've done, what's been done to you." The enemy has come to steal our hope — to rob us of our self-worth and keep us feeling useless.

But there is also a vote cast over us that is a vote of truth: We are mighty overcomers who have been given a hope and a future.

Each one of us has the deciding vote. We break the tie. With whom will we side? Let us vote for truth!

To succeed in any lifestyle change, we must draw upon God's power. He wants to renew our minds and show us His perspective. He works progressively over time. As we wait for Him to work, He gives us power to transform. His desire is for us to "prosper in all things and be in health" (3 John 2, NKJV).

PART FIVE

FOOD
FOR LIFE,
FOREVER

TWENTY

GETTING
THE
VISION

IS THERE SOMETHING you can do to make your life better — or worse? If you answered yes to this question, you have taken a step toward taking responsibility for your life and your future. Yesterday ended last night. We have to choose what we will do with our today.

This is the day to slip gently into a healthier way of eating without starving yourself or running yourself ragged. Just decide today to turn from the path of confusion and take a small step on the road to looking and feeling better.

Choose to eat well of the food that gives life. Food is the perfect fuel designed to meet the needs of your body — the perfect source of nourishment to keep your body working for you.

Our bodies can walk in wellness — full of energy, thinking clearly, managing stress — if we feed them the right thing at the right time. And that means we must trust that the return on our investment will be worth our effort, that eating won't make us gain weight improperly or get out of control. We have to get beyond the fear of food.

It does take planning. Vending machines don't stock the healthiest of foods. Along with planning, we must remember that the best plans don't always work out as we hope. We don't have total control over every aspect of our lives, and that's good. We've not been called to control anything — except the choices we make.

You have been designed to accomplish, engineered to succeed and empowered to achieve greatness. Don't let any life trap hinder you another second.

Change has its challenges. Expect stress, sabotages and setbacks. But keep your eyes lifted up to the vision of living life well. You deserve the best!

⌣ NOTES ⌣

Chapter Two:
Making Peace With Food

1. Paul Ernsberger, "The Death of Dieting," *American Health* (January/February 1985), pp. 29-33.
2. From a report released in March 1992 by a National Institutes of Health panel on weight-loss programs (as reported by Sally Squires in the *Washington Post* and reprinted in the *Orlando Sentinel,* June 9, 1992).

Chapter Five:
Eating Is Better Than Starving:
Eat Early and Eat Often

1. The Vanderbilt study cited was mentioned in the October 1992 issue of *Men's Health* magazine (Emmaus, Pa.: Rodale Press), p. 41.

Chapter Six:
Eating Is Better Than Starving:
Eat Balanced and Eat Lean

1. A 1988 study directed by Darlene Dreon at Stanford University, "Dietary Fat: Carbohydrate Ratio and Obesity Ratio in Middle-aged Men," found that the percentage of body fat in the participants was directly related to the proportion of their daily calories derived from fat, not to their total calories. A study from Harvard Medical School completed in the fall of 1993 came to the same conclusion. In 141 women studied, excess weight was linked to fat consumption, independent of calorie intake. The disease linkage has been shown in numerous other ongoing studies as well, including one by the U.S. Department of Health and Human Services, 1989; a study by the Multiple Risk Factor Intervention Trial Research Group (M.R.F.I.T.), as reported in the article "MortalityRates After 10.5 Years for Participants in the M.R.F.I.T.," *Journal of the American Medical Association* (JAMA), 1990, 263:1795-1801; and in *The Framingham Study:*

The Epidemiology of Atherosclerotic Disease, T. R. Dawber (Cambridge, Mass.: Harvard University Press, 1980).
2. *Diet, Nutrition and Cancer,* 1982, a landmark report by a special panel of the National Academy of Sciences.

Chapter Nine:
Stress Is a Stretch That Will Make You Snap or Make You Strong!

1. R. S. Eliot and D. L. Breo, *Is It Worth Dying For?* (New York: Bantam Books, 1986).
2. J. Kiecolt-Glaser and R. Glaser, "Major Life Changes, Chronic Stress, and Immunity," *Adv Biochem Psychopharmacol,* 1988; 44:217-24.
3. P. Ekman, R. W. Levenson and W. V. Friesen, "Autonomic Nervous System Activity Distinguishes Among Emotions," *Science,* 1983; 221(4616):1208-10; Eliot and Breo, 1986; Kiecolt-Glaser and Glaser, 1988.
4. K. L. Lichstein, "Everyday, Low-Level Tension Can Kill Us," *Bottom Line,* 15 February 1993, p. 11; Eliot and Breo, 1986; Kiecolt-Glaser and Glaser, 1988; Ekman, Levenson and Friesen, 1983.
5. Lydia Temoshok, Ph.D., *The Type C Connection: The Behavioral Links to Cancer and Your Health* (New York: Random House, 1992); Eliot and Breo, 1986; Kiecolt-Glaser and Glaser, 1988; Ekman, Levenson and Friesen, 1983.
6. Reported in the August 1994 issue of *Men's Health* magazine.

Chapter Ten:
Exercise Is Vital to Well-Being

1. The research information in this chapter was taken from the following sources:
S. N. Blair, H. W. Kohl, R. S. Paffenbarger, et al., "Physical Fitness and All-Cause Mortality," *Journal of the American Medical Association* (JAMA), 1989, 262:2395-2401.
B. Epstein, "Higher Resistance," *Men's Fitness,* May 1993.
J. M. Rippe, A. Ward, H. P. Porcari, and P. S. Freedson, "Walking for Health and Fitness," *Journal of the American Medical Association,* 1988, 259:2720-24.
Vic Sussman, "No Pain and Lots of Gain," *U.S. News & World Report,* May 4, 1992, pp. 86-88.
S. R. Yarnall, "F.I.T. to a T," *Stay Well, America,* 1990, vol. 4.

Chapter Eleven:
Rest Is the Key to Recharging

1. C. Ferrari, "Guide to Energy: The Sleep Factor," *McCall's*, August 1991, p. 32.
2. R. Cartwright, *Crisis Dreaming* (New York: HarperCollins, 1991).
3. A 1992 report from the National Commission on Sleep Disorders Research.
4. Ibid.
5. R. Cartwright, "All About Sleep," *Bottom Line*, 30 September 1992.

Chapter Fifteen:
Overcoming Sabotage

1. Cheryl McCall, "The Cruelest Crime — Sexual Abuse of Children: The Victims, the Offenders, How to Protect Your Family," *Life*, December 1984, p. 35.

Chapter Eighteen:
Looking Back

1. K. Halni, J. Fallk and E. Schwartz, "Binge Eating and Vomiting," *Psychological Medicine*, November 1981, n (4): 697-706; H. G. Pope and J. I. Hudson, "Prevalence of Anorexia Nervosa in the Student Population," *International Journal of Eating Disorders*, 1984, 4:45-53.
2. Hilde Bruch, *Eating Disorders: Obesity, Anorexia Nervosa and the Person Within* (New York: Basic Books, 1973).

✌ RECIPE INDEX ✌

OTHER BOOKS AND TAPES

BY PAMELA M. SMITH, R.D.

Eat Well—Live Well

BESTSELLER! This is Pam's nutrition guidebook for healthy and productive living. This large, deluxe hardback edition presents "The Ten Commandments of Good Nutrition" in detail, along with giving directions for menu planning, grocery shopping, and dining out, from fast food to gourmet. The large cookbook section contains innovative recipes that can be prepared in a time-saving manner. Meal plans for weight loss and weight management are included. This is a "must have" book for personal and family nutrition. (Creation House)

The Good Life—A Healthy Cookbook

The wonderful feast of Pam's most savory recipes. This deluxe hardback edition features full color photography in a "coffee-table style" presentation. Complete meals, with all of the trimmings, for breakfast, lunch, and dinner, plus scrumptious desserts and power snacks, are detailed. Quick-cooking techniques and plate design are presented in an easy and beautiful way. For the novice or gourmet cook, this book is designed for everyone to enjoy. (Creation House)

Food For Life

BESTSELLER! More than a guide and cookbook, *Food For Life* shows you how to eat smart and walk in abundant life. It presents Pam's "Seven Secrets for Staying Fit, Fueled, and Free"—helping you to explore your relationship with food and yourself. Discover how to choose food wisely, manage weight, and develop a proper perspective for nourishing yourself physically, emotionally, and spiritually. Meal plans, recipes, and specific action plans are detailed. Available in deluxe hardback and softcover editions. (Creation House)

Food For Life—One Day at a Time

This thirty-day devotional guide will equip you and empower you to break free of the Food Trap—forever! A perfect accompaniment for the book, *Food For Life*. (Creation House)

Healthy Expectations

This is the expectant mother's handbook with the latest information for nourishing mom and baby. It includes an extensive question-and-answer section with a proven, natural technique for overcoming morning sickness. This book is filled with love and wisdom, meal plans, and tips for direction before, during, and after delivery. (Creation House)

Healthy Expectations—Devotional Journal

A beautiful accompaniment for the expectant mother, this devotional embraces the truth and wonder of the "life" residing within her. Reading, meditating, and reflecting on God's Word will bring a "peace for the process" that nourishes body, soul, and spirit. Record the thoughts, impressions, and memories in this lovely journal. (Creation House)

Alive and Well in the Fast Lane

This fun and lighthearted nutritional guidebook is for the whole family—especially teens. It is published in a whimsical, handwritten, and illustrated style that really hits home with humor. Includes recipes and the "Ten Commandments of Healthy Eating" on the run. (Not in Bookstores—Direct Purchase Only)

Come Cook With Me

Hooray for the kid's cookbook! This book shows how to teach children nutrition by teaching them how to cook healthfully. It is great for "picky eaters" and includes kid-proven recipes, kitchen safety, and some great tips on manners. Handwritten and fun, this book is a favorite of young chefs. (Not in Bookstores—Direct Purchase Only)

AUDIO AND VIDEO TAPES

The Seven Secrets for Living the Good Life (Series)

In this dynamic four-tape series, Pam will teach you how to blend healthy living into your busy schedule, turbo-charge your metabolism and immune systems, seal your "energy leaks," and recharge and refuel while you "lean" down. Pam will also demonstrate her delicious and healthy cooking techniques that you can do, along with tips for traveling and how to dine out healthfully. These are fun and incredibly informative. Available in audio or video formats. (Not in Bookstores—Direct Purchase Only)

The Food Trap Seminar (Book and Tape Package)

In this dynamic series, you will hear Pam present a live seminar asking the question "Is the Refrigerator Light the Light of Your Life?" Informative and enlightening, this four-tape audio series, including *The Food Trap* book, reveals case studies and personal insights into the physical, emotional, and spiritual implications of food dependencies. You will learn techniques for breaking free and living free in all these areas of life. (Not in Bookstores—Direct Purchase Only)

Other Individual Tape Titles Available

SPECIAL OFFER

BY PAMELA M. SMITH, R.D.
FREE!

"Exceptional Energy"
Audiocassette Tape

For a free copy of Pamela Smith's "Exceptional Energy"
audio tape, please complete and mail the following coupon
(plus U.S. $2.50 to cover postage and handling).

❏ Please send me a free copy of Pamela Smith's
"Exceptional Energy" audiocassette tape.
I have enclosed U.S. $2.50 to cover postage and handling.
(Canadian residents, please enclose U.S. $3.50).

❏ Please send me a free Food Diary.

❏ Please send me information on your Newsletter.

Name ....

Address ....

City/State/Zip ....

Please send coupon and check to:

PAMELA M. SMITH, R.D.
P.O. Box 541009 ❖ Orlando, FL 32854-1009

FOR MORE INFORMATION

on Pamela Smith's books, tapes, speaking
and seminar/workshops, please write or call:

Pamela M. Smith, R.D.
P.O. Box 541009
Orlando, FL 32854

(800) 896-4010 (orders)
(407) 855-8630 (information)

or

Creation House
600 Rinehart Road
Lake Mary, FL 32746

(800) 283-8494
(800) 283-4561 (fax)

Please send Pam your stories and victories at:

E-mail: PS4Health@aol.com

PAMELA M. SMITH, R.D., L.D.N.

P AMELA M. SMITH is a nationally known nutritionist, best-selling author and culinary consultant. She has been featured on *The Today Show, CNN News, The 700 Club, Focus on the Family,* and a number of nationally broadcast radio talk shows.

Pamela is the founder of Nutritional Counseling Services in Orlando, Florida, one of the original private practices of dietetics in America. She is the nutritionist for the Orlando Magic NBA team and for individual players and other professional athletes nationwide. She has also served as consultant to industry giants such as Walt Disney World and Hyatt Hotels and Resorts and is the director of culinary development for General Mills Restaurants, New Business Division.

Pamela counsels her clients on an interactive basis, helping them to identify and alter eating and behavioral habits for disease prevention; peak performance in sports; child and family nutrition; weight loss; dining-out strategies; and, very important, stress and emotional implications.

Her books include *Eat Well—Live Well,* a best-selling nutritional guide and cookbook; *Alive and Well in the Fast Lane,* a lighthearted book with the Ten Commandments of Good Nutrition; *Perfectly Pregnant,* a nutrition book for the expectant mother; *Come Cook With Me,* an extraordinary children's cookbook; and *Food For Life,* an in-depth look at the physical, emotional, and spiritual aspects of nourishing our bodies.

She received her degree in nutrition from Florida State University and completed her American Dietetic Association internship at Miami-Valley Hospital in Dayton, Ohio. She has completed continuing education at the Cooper Clinic in Dallas, Texas, as well as through the Harvard Medical School. She was also the nutrition instructor at the University of Central Florida, Department of Nursing.

Pamela has received the Recognized Young Dietitian award for the State of Florida as well as the Award for Excellence in medical journalism by the Florida branch of the American Medical Association. She has been featured on radio and TV talk and news shows since 1980 and is in demand for corporate, top-management programs, seminars, conventions, and corporate wellness programs.